The All-Natural
Cardio Cure

The All-Natural Cardio Cure

A DRUG-FREE CHOLESTEROL AND CARDIAC INFLAMMATION REDUCTION PROGRAM

Allan Magaziner, D.O.
with
Batya Swift Yasgur, M.A., MSW

AVERY
a member of Penguin Group (USA) Inc.
New York

Neither the publisher nor the authors are engaged in rendering professional advice or services to the individual reader. The ideas, procedures, and suggestions contained in this book are not intended as a substitute for consulting with your physician. All matters regarding health require medical supervision. Neither the authors nor the publisher shall be liable or responsible for any loss, injury, or damage allegedly arising from any information or suggestion in this book. The opinions expressed in this book represent the personal views of the authors and not of the publisher.

While the authors have made every effort to provide accurate telephone numbers and Internet addresses at the time of publication, neither the publisher nor the authors assume any responsibility for errors or for changes that occur after publication.

Most Avery books are available at special quantity discounts for bulk purchase for sales promotions, premiums, fund-raising, and educational needs. Special books or book excerpts also can be created to fit specific needs. For details, write Penguin Group (USA) Inc. Special Markets, 375 Hudson Street, New York 10014.

a member of
Penguin Group (USA) Inc.
375 Hudson Street
New York, NY 10014
www.penguin.com

Copyright © 2004 by Allan Magaziner
All rights reserved. This books, or parts thereof, may not be reproduced in any form without permission. Published simultaneously in Canada

Library of Congress Cataloging-in-Publication Data

Magaziner, Allan.
The all-natural cardio cure : a drug-free cholesterol and cardiac inflammation reduction program / Allan Magaziner, with Batya Swift Yasgur.
p. cm.
Includes bibliographical references and index.
ISBN 1-58333-179-4
1. Heart—Diseases—Prevention—Popular works.   2. Cardiovascular system—Diseases—Prevention—Popular works.   I. Yasgur, Batya Swift. II. Title.
RC672.M34   2004   2003062807
616.1'05—dc22

Printed in the United States of America
1 3 5 7 9 10 8 6 4 2

BOOK DESIGN BY MEIGHAN CAVANAUGH

The spirit and devotion of both my parents
inspire me in all aspects of my life.

I dedicate this book to them
with gratitude and love.

Acknowledgments

I would like to begin by thanking my mentors, who have influenced my thinking in all areas of medicine and whose perspectives have ultimately led to the writing of this book. In particular, Paul Ridker, M.D., and Kilmer McCully, M.D., both of whom addressed the American College for Advancement in Medicine (ACAM), had a profound impact on my approach to cardiovascular disease. Their groundbreaking research opened new vistas, and they have both made significant inroads in medical understanding of atherosclerosis and cardiovascular disease. Jonathan Wright, M.D., and Jeffrey Bland, Ph.D., opened my eyes to the importance of nutritional biochemistry and dietary supplementation in all areas of illness and health, including cardiovascular disease.

Writing a book can be daunting and challenging at times. I would like to thank those who have helped me in the process of preparing this book for publication. Tamar Messer is a gifted artist whose illustrations have enhanced this book. Many thanks to Shoshana Thaler for her careful work in preparing the references. And of course, thanks to Batya Swift Yasgur, M.A., MSW, for her tireless labor, invaluable input, and commitment to seeing this project through to completion; and for her friendship and support.

Thanks to my hardworking office staff for their encouragement, and of course to all my patients, who have taught me as much as I have taught them. This book is for all of you—it could not have been written without you.

Last but not least, thanks to my lovely wife, Suzanne, for all her moral support, encouragement, and excellent insights and advice. She served as an extremely helpful sounding board throughout this project. And to my wonderful children, who often had to entertain themselves while their daddy was busy writing. You guys are the best!

Contents

Introduction   *1*

PART ONE: What Is My Risk?
An Expanding Understanding of Risk Factors

1. The Heart of the Matter   *7*

2. The Doctor Says My Cholesterol Is Too High   *18*

3. Additional Clues in the Blood   *36*

4. High Blood Pressure: The "Silent" Killer   *47*

5. Diabetes and Cardiovascular Disease: Making the Link   *53*

6. Obesity: Not Just a Cosmetic Problem   *61*

7. Your Heart Goes Up in Smoke   *69*

8. Other Risk Factors for Cardiovascular Disease   *74*

9. Assessing Your Risk   *81*

PART TWO: What Can I Do?
The DEAR Program

10. Eating with CARE: Basic Elements of the Diet — *91*

11. Customizing the CARE Diet — *141*

12. Supplements That Care for Your Heart — *171*

13. Exercise: A Great Cholesterol-Buster — *206*

14. Caring for Your Heart: Stress Reduction — *224*

15. Obstacles to Self-Care — *246*

16. DEAR Diary: Your Personal Workbook — *256*

17. Conclusions — *270*

Glossary — *273*

Suggestions for Further Reading — *279*

Selected References — *283*

Resources — *291*

Index — *299*

Introduction

Cardiovascular disease is the leading cause of illness and death in the United States. It accounts for half a million deaths per year and causes an annual expenditure of $200 billion. It is the most prevalent epidemic in this country . . . and also the most preventable.

In my medical practice, I specialize in nutritional and natural approaches, and about one-quarter of my patients suffer from one form or other of cardiovascular disease. Many of my patients consult me after being treated by conventionally oriented physicians. Some have already had surgical procedures, such as angioplasty ("ballooning") or bypass surgery. And almost all of my patients with high cholesterol have been treated with pharmaceutical therapy, usually with a class of drugs called *statins*. Unfortunately, many report that the side effects of their medication are as bad as the illness itself.

To help the millions of people who suffer from high cholesterol and are seeking alternatives to statin drugs, I decided to develop a special program. However, my program is aimed not only at people with elevated cholesterol levels, but people who suffer from a group of other conditions as well. Although it is still seen as extremely dangerous, high cholesterol is no longer regarded as the single major risk factor for the development of cardiovascular disease. Rather, it is one of a network of common risk factors that often intersect, creating a condition known as *metabolic syndrome,* or *syndrome X*. Scientists now know that individuals with syndrome X are in great danger, and they are seeking to aggressively address this condition.

The identification of syndrome X is an enormous step in the understanding of cardiovascular disease. But it raises a question: What ties this apparently disparate group of symptoms into a unified "syndrome"? The answer lies in an exciting new area of discovery and research: inflammation.

Scientists have recently come to understand that elevated cholesterol, hypertension, and the other components of syndrome X all contribute to inflammation in the arteries; and it is inflammation that turns out to be the primary culprit in CVD.

But there is a downside to this research. The wonderful changes and discoveries that are rocking the world of cardiovascular disease research are resulting in a serious potential problem—the overprescription of statin drugs. The NCEP-ATP III guidelines that lower the cholesterol threshold mean that an increasing number of people will be seen as having abnormally high cholesterol levels and will be given treatment, most likely with statin drugs.

The good news is that there are safe and effective alternatives to statin drugs for reducing both cholesterol *and* inflammation. In fact, the emerging research into the role of inflammation in heart disease has bolstered my commitment to these alternatives.

The Evolution of the DEAR Program

In medical school, I was privileged to attend a presentation on mind-body medicine given by Bernie Siegel, M.D. This awakened my interest in holistic approaches to health. I became increasingly interested in nutrition and natural supplements and became increasingly appreciative of the role of mind and spirit in physical processes. By the time I had completed my training, I was familiar with holistic approaches and began to incorporate them into my practice. I have been recommending my DEAR program to patients for nearly twenty years, and I know that it is effective. New research has lent extra scientific validity to my approach and has shed light on why my program works, not only to lower cholesterol but also to reduce the overall risk of cardiovascular disease.

This book describes my program, which I affectionately call DEAR:

- *D*iet
- *E*xercise
- *A*dditional supplementation
- *R*elaxation

I like this name because I believe that to be successful in implementing this program, you must love yourself. Please understand that the self-love I'm talking about is not selfishness. Rather, it is a beautiful and necessary part of human survival, as individuals and as a species. It also involves loving others and accepting others' love. It lies at the heart of all holistic medicine and involves nurturing the body, mind, and spirit with healthy food, exercise, and supplements or medications when necessary, as well as with intellectual, emotional, and spiritual forms of expansion, stimulation, relaxation, and fun. I break down these health components throughout the book to help you achieve your goals.

Part 1 of this book discusses risk factors for the development of cardiovascular disease, including high cholesterol, high triglycerides, diabetes, and high blood pressure. It will help you understand why smoking is a dangerous activity not only for your lungs but also for your heart and why obesity is a health hazard, not merely a cosmetic problem. This section also provides you with the tools you need to assess your own risk level, which will enable you to personalize your treatment. In part 2, I lay out my program and help you customize it to fit your current state of health and your lifestyle. There are also worksheets to help you organize your new lifestyle. At the back of the book, you will find a glossary, suggestions for further reading, and a list of helpful resources. (Note that this is only a partial list; you can access a more complete list on my website, www.allnaturalcardiocure.com).

    I hope that you come to realize how dear you are to yourself and to others, and that you deserve to give yourself the best tender loving care.

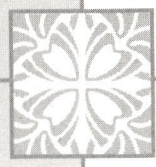

PART ONE

What Is My Risk?

An Expanding Understanding
of Risk Factors

 The Heart of the Matter

My crown is in my heart.
—William Shakespeare

... who has fashioned human beings with wisdom and created within them openings and channels. It is known before Your throne of glory that if one of these should inappropriately open or inappropriately close, it would be impossible to survive.
—Jewish prayer

Think of how much attention we focus on the heart.

It fills our poetry and our metaphor. When we are sad, we are "heartsick." When we are bereaved, we are "heartbroken." When we want someone to have compassion, we say, "Have a heart." A sincere statement is "heartfelt." Our beloved is our "heartthrob," we thank people from the "bottom of our heart," and the center of an issue is the "heart of the matter."

The heart occupies more than metaphoric significance in common parlance. When we're upset, our heart "skips a beat" or "stands still." When we're angry, we say, "You're giving me heart failure." No medical term is more dreaded than "heart attack."

Considering how important the heart is in our society, we don't take very good care of it. Despite extensive campaigns by the American Heart Association and other organizations, diseases of the heart and circulatory system are still the number one cause of death in the United

States, as well as in Europe and Asia. These conditions, which are known collectively as *cardiovascular disease* (CVD), account for 1 million deaths in the United States every year and are responsible for 40 percent of all deaths in this country. This translates into one death every thirty-three seconds, or 2,600 people each day! We all are terrified of cancer—rightly so—but nearly twice as many people die from CVD than cancer.

In addition, according to the World Health Organization (WHO), CVD is responsible for an estimated 17 million deaths worldwide each year. It is also responsible for a staggering amount of disability and impairment. For example, the American Heart Association estimates that in the year 2002 alone, $330 billion of health costs, including health expenditures and lost productivity, were attributable to cardiovascular disease. CVD can thus be seen as one of the most menacing forces at large on the planet.

What causes a heart attack or stroke? The simplest answer—and the view maintained by scientists for many decades—is that it results in blood flow to and from the heart being either partially or completely obstructed. Due to the buildup of a substance called *plaque,* the available space for blood flow is limited. It takes the blood longer to move through the narrowed opening. Moreover, the walls of the blood vessels are not as elastic and flexible as they should be. The accumulated plaque stiffens them, so they do not expand properly to allow blood to pass through. This is *atherosclerosis.*

When this happens, several possible consequences can ensue. Oxygen-rich blood might not reach the heart, leading to the death of heart tissue, a situation known as *myocardial infarction,* or heart attack; or it might not reach the brain, leading to a *cerebral vascular accident,* or stroke. A blood clot can travel through the blood vessels, lodging itself in the heart or brain, causing similar damage. Additionally, blood flow to vital organs such as the kidneys and lungs becomes impaired.

A vicious cycle ensues, because the heart starts to work harder to pump blood through the body and compensate for the inefficient blood flow. This increases the blood pressure—another significant risk factor for the development of CVD. And, of course, because the heart itself is working harder, it is experiencing more stress and strain than it should.

Cholesterol is the first problematic substance in the blood that is associated with the risk of developing CVD. Historically, it is the oldest known risk factor that is measurable by blood tests, and much research has gone into establishing guidelines and creating treatment protocols—some of them helpful, others problematic. It is also the first word that jumps to mind when we think of blood and CVD. But cholesterol isn't the only risk factor measurable by blood tests. And the plaque associated with atherosclerosis is emerging as a problem with more dimensions and facets than originally thought.

Inflammation: The Body's Defender Becomes Its Attacker

Scientists have begun looking at another factor for CVD—inflammation. When a foreign substance enters your bloodstream due to an infection or injury, the cells in your immune system go to work, engulfing the invader, gobbling it up, carting off the debris, and sealing off the injury to allow healing to begin. In addition, a reaction known as the inflammatory response takes place. For a localized injury, this response typically causes an array of symptoms, including swelling, redness, heat, and sometimes itching. If the body is fighting a virus or bacteria, the person may experience fever, pain, and chills.

Without this process, every little germ floating through our environment could be a potential killer. So, immune cells are crucial for our survival and our health—when they are present in the proper balance.

The Progression to Blocked Arteries

Scientists used to think that cardiovascular disease resulted simply from too much cholesterol clogging the arteries. Now we realize that this model is overly simplistic and that other substances and processes also contribute. Cholesterol combines with cellular waste products, calcium, and other substances to form plaque along the arterial walls. That plaque is destructive because it is caused by an inflammatory process and, in turn, leads to further inflammation. Following is a summary of what happens.

DAMAGE TO THE ENDOTHELIUM

The *endothelium* is a layer of cells that covers the entire inner structure of the blood vessel. The endothelium can become damaged by factors such as high blood pressure, certain infections and viruses, environmental toxins, heavy metals, and elevated levels of substances such as *homocysteine*. These factors combine to attack the endothelium. If damaged, the endothelium becomes permeable, or porous. Instead of being smooth, as a healthy endothelium should be, it has tiny openings.

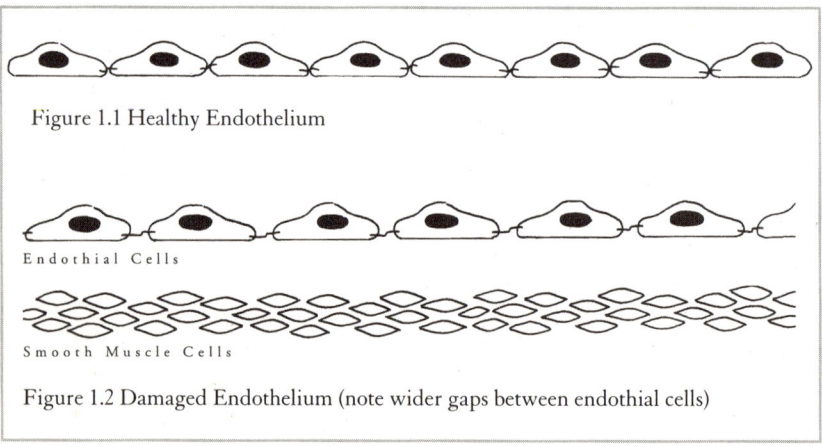

Figure 1.1 Healthy Endothelium

Endothial Cells

Smooth Muscle Cells

Figure 1.2 Damaged Endothelium (note wider gaps between endothial cells)

INFILTRATION OF THE ENDOTHELIUM BY CIRCULATING FAT

If there is too much fat in the bloodstream, it will accumulate on the arterial walls. A fatty deposit on the endothelium is a major irritant to this delicate surface. In a properly functioning body, the fatty deposits would be vanquished due to the smoothness of the endothelium (it's harder for the cells to remain attached to a smooth surface) and to the fact that immune cells engulf and cart away the unwanted fat cells. But when the endothelium has already been damaged, it is no longer smooth. It is permeable, so it is unable to sustain the onslaught of additional fat cells, which proceed to worm their way into the openings in the endothelium. The body then perceives this as an injury, and the immune system rushes in to vanquish the invaders and heal the injury. Unfortunately, the immune system's well-intentioned attempts at healing often cause further damage.

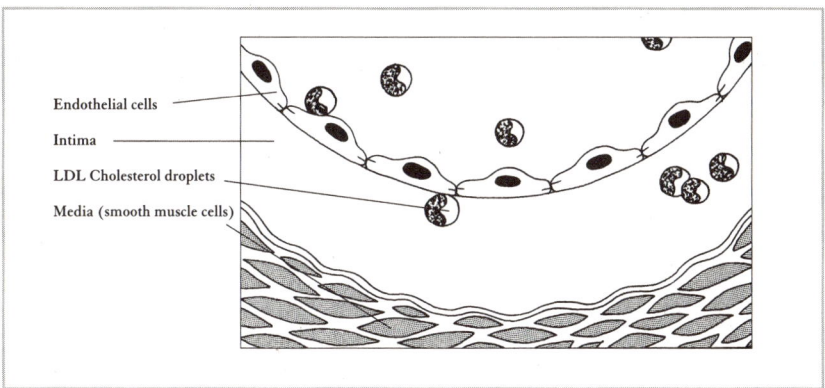

Figure 1.3 Invasion of the Fat Cells

OVERZEALOUS MACROPHAGES

In the case of a routine injury, scavenger cells called *macrophages* trap and engulf invading cells and consume them. Once this has been accomplished, other cells such as *leukocytes* (white blood cells) carry away the macrophages so that they, together with their destructive cargo, do not remain within the body to cause more damage. But when there is a large volume of fat-filled macrophages—called *foam cells*—the leukocytes cannot meet the challenge. They stay within the area, forming what is known as a *fatty streak*, which is the earliest sign of an atherosclerotic plaque.

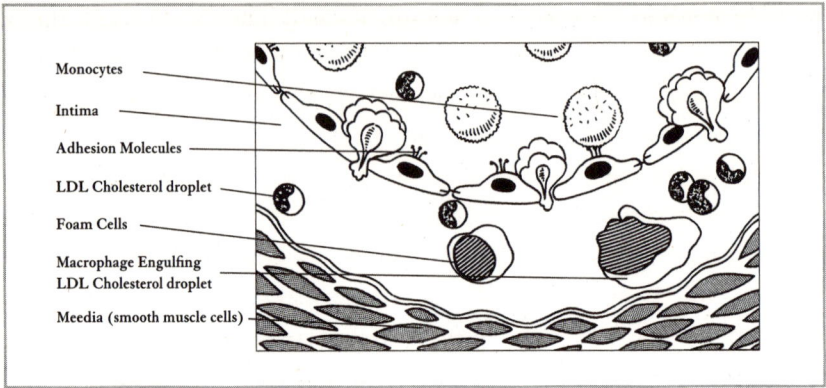

Figure 1.4 Macrophages Engulfing LDL Cholesterol to Form Foam Cells

THE FORMATION OF A FATTY STREAK

The *lesion* (the general medical word for an injury or localized abnormality) filled with many foam cells that is called a fatty streak typically grows because the immune cells, such as leukocytes and macrophages, multiply inside the lesion. This in turn gives rise to a flurry of activity and an influx of numerous pro-inflammatory substances of all kinds. All of this has the effect of increasing the stickiness of the endothelial wall and making it even more permeable to leukocytes, monocytes, and LDL cholesterol, which continue to enter and burrow inside the lesion.

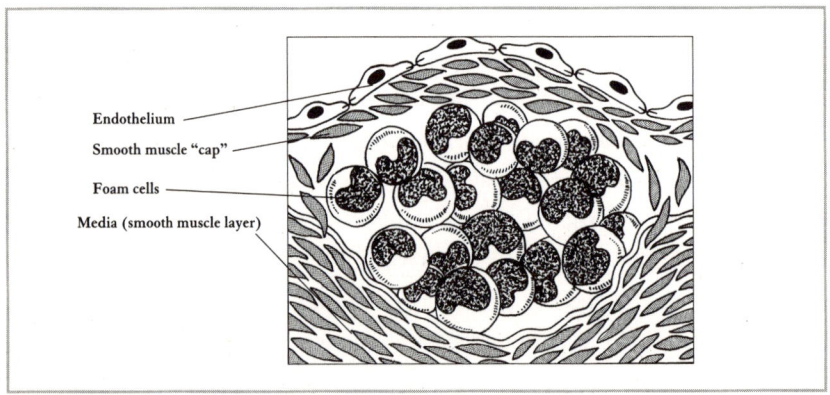

Figure 1.5 Plaque Lesion

Then, other immune cells are summoned. They arrive with the intention of healing or sealing the injury. Platelets in particular become sticky around the site of an injury and play a crucial role in the formation of blood clots. (In fact, the mechanism of blood-thinning medications makes the platelets less sticky.) But the sticky platelets invite more oxidized LDL cholesterol to stick to the site, and the lesion continues to grow. (*Oxidized cholesterol* forms when cholesterol undergoes a chemical reaction with oxygen, creating a new and dangerous compound.) As the lesion grows, more and more naturally occurring chemical messengers called *cytokines* are released, and the area becomes even stickier—a truly vicious cycle.

THE MIGRATION OF SMOOTH MUSCLE CELLS TO COVER THE LESION

Realizing that it cannot vanquish the lesion, the body's next attempt to heal the injury is to seal it off. A tough, fibrous covering is formed on the foam cells, often called the *fibrous cap*. It seals off the lesion to prevent further damage.

Under the cap, a nasty brew of foam cells, leukocytes, and cellular debris simmers, caused by *apoptosis* (the death of cells) and *necrosis* (decay triggered by the death of tissues). Normally, dead cells are replaced by new cells. But when the cells under the fibrous cap die, they cannot be replaced or discarded because they are sealed in, so they decay, leaving what is called a *necrotic core*. The entire structure—the cap and the destructive substances contained beneath it—is called an *advanced, complicated atherosclerotic lesion*. These lesions are the building blocks of plaque.

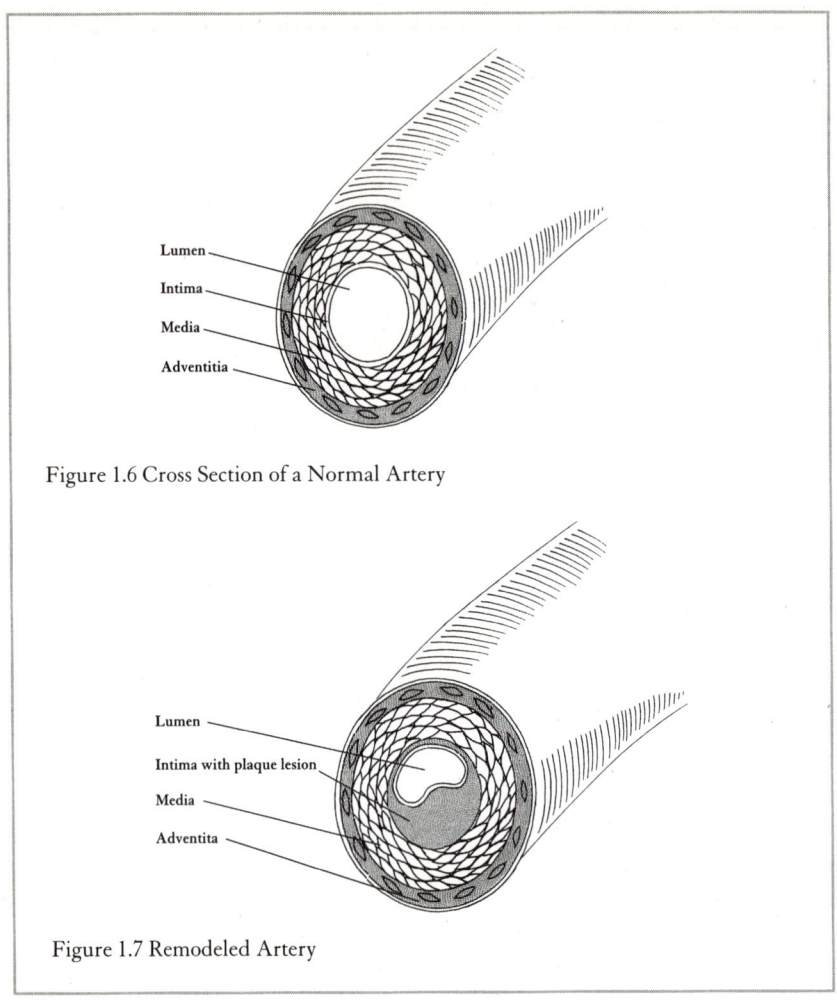

Figure 1.6 Cross Section of a Normal Artery

Figure 1.7 Remodeled Artery

REMODELING OF THE ARTERY TO ACCOMMODATE PLAQUE BUILDUP

As long as the lesion remains small and confined, the artery—whose walls are elastic and quite flexible—can expand to accommodate the capped foam cells. Scientists call this process *remodeling*. But if the lesion becomes too big or if many lesions start to accumulate, the artery cannot sufficiently reshape itself. The *lumen* (the channel within the blood vessel through which the blood flows) begins to narrow, and the arterial walls lose their elasticity.

WHAT HAPPENS NEXT—TWO SCENARIOS

At this point, we know that there are significant plaque deposits in various stages of development along the arteries. We do not know, however, whether this person will go on to have a heart attack or stroke. How can we find out?

There are two scenarios to explore. In the first, the person is less likely to suffer from heart attack or stroke, although he or she may have other symptoms of coronary artery disease. In the second scenario, he or she is at great risk for having a heart attack or stroke.

Scenario 1: Stable Plaque

If the person begins leading a heart-healthy lifestyle, the toxins and inflammatory substances in the bloodstream can drop significantly. There won't be anything to disturb the fibrous cap, and it could remain stable and solid, perhaps for decades.

This does not mean that the person is healthy or guaranteed never to suffer a heart attack. For one thing, the arteries are still hardened and constricted, and the heart must still work much harder than it should to pump blood through vessels that are narrower than they should be and refuse to expand. This can lead to a condition known as *angina pectoris*—chest pains commonly associated with heart disease. If arteries in the leg are affected, the person may experience numbness, fatigue, or pain in his legs, especially when walking. This is called *intermittent claudication*.

In addition, atherosclerosis—even with stable plaque—can lead to a heart attack. Surprisingly, though, this dynamic is responsible for relatively few heart attacks—only 15 percent! Many people live to ripe ages with high levels of cholesterol and arteries encrusted with stable plaque.

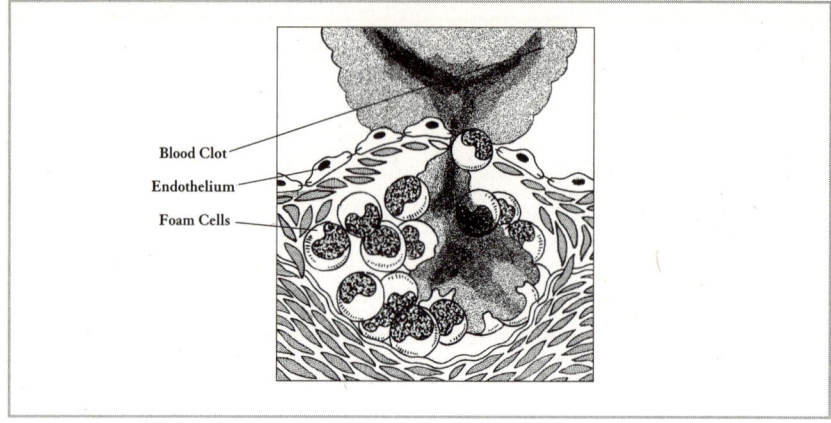

Figure 1.8 Rupture of the Fibrous Cap

Scenario 2: Vulnerable (Unstable) Plaque

Another possibility is that the fibrous cap continues to erode as a result of the ongoing inflammatory assault, and the lesion continues to swell. Eventually, the cap ruptures, releasing a cloud of noxious, rapidly clotting substances into the bloodstream. A blood clot, or *thrombus,* is formed. If the thrombus lodges itself in a coronary artery and blocks it, the result is a heart attack. If it travels to the brain and lodges itself there, the result is a stroke. With this scenario, it doesn't matter what size the original lesion was—small lesions are as dangerous as large ones.

Scientists estimate that rupture of vulnerable plaque might be responsible for most heart attacks, especially in people in their forties and fifties. Even worse, these heart attacks are more likely to be fatal. Some researchers have looked at the correlation between white blood cell count, which suggests the presence of a high-level inflammatory response, and the incidence of death following a heart attack. These researchers found that patients with the highest white blood cell counts had the greatest risk of death. They also had poorer responses to blood-thinning treatments. These findings support the growing body of evidence suggesting that inflammation is a prime culprit in the development of cardiovascular disease.

Conditions Associated with Cardiovascular Disease

Heart attack and stroke are the two most dangerous outcomes of atherosclerotic plaque and cardiovascular disease. However, there are other cardiac illnesses, less dramatic but also serious, that can result from plaque buildup and endothelial dysfunction:

- Angina, which occurs when the blood supply to the heart does not meet the heart's needs and causes chest pain that typically increases with activity and lessens with rest;
- Congestive heart failure, which occurs if the heart does not pump adequate amounts of blood out into the body, causing fluid buildup in the lungs and, sometimes, the ankles or legs, as well as shortness of breath and fatigue;
- Peripheral artery disease, or hardening of the arteries in the leg, which can cause foot or leg pain, cramping, or heaviness that increases with effort and vanishes when you stand still;
- Valvular heart disease, which occurs if any of the four heart valves that separate the four chambers of the heart leaks, potentially leading to symptoms including shortness of breath, especially with exertion; chest pain or discomfort; chronic cough; and general fatigue.

It would be easy to know that you are in danger of such problems if you could see the interior of your blood vessels and observe their blocked and inflamed state. In real life, however, it is not so easy to assess the extent and type of damage along blood vessel walls. In chapter 2, we will look at diagnostic tools that provide essential clues to an individual's risk of developing cardiovascular disease.

2 The Doctor Says My Cholesterol Is Too High

Our wasted oil unprofitably burns...
—William Cowper

I'm sure you have heard of cholesterol. It has become a household word, thanks to hard work on the part of the American Heart Association. We see it in countless television commercials and encounter it as we browse through supermarket aisles—this or that product is touted as virtuous because it is "low in cholesterol" or because it will "lower your cholesterol." It seems like a new study on cholesterol comes out every other day, with foods that were once considered detrimental suddenly praised as being healthful, and vice versa. *Cholesterol* is probably as common a word as *blood* or *heart*. But in my experience, few people actually know what cholesterol is or why it's bad for the heart. So let me introduce you to this ubiquitous but little-understood substance.

Cholesterol is an odorless, white, waxy substance that is made in our bodies. Although it is present in many of the foods we eat, it is actually primarily manufactured in the liver. Only a third of the cholesterol in our bodies, on average, comes from diet alone. So even if you are a strict vegetarian who has never eaten a bite of cholesterol-containing food, your liver would still produce a measurable quantity of this substance from fats found in other foods that you eat. Other sites for the synthesis of cholesterol are the adrenal glands and the reproductive organs, but the liver does the lion's share of the work.

Cholesterol is a *lipid,* or fatty substance. And although it has become virtually a dirty word in American parlance, that's really unfair. Having some cholesterol in our bodies is not only beneficial but actually necessary for our health. Cholesterol helps to insulate the nerves. Your nerves are like electric wires running through your body. Like the electric wires in your house, your nerves need insulation, and this is provided by cholesterol. Cholesterol is also the building block of the sex hormones—estrogen, progesterone, and testosterone—which play a crucial role in the reproductive cycle of both men and women. Cholesterol is also instrumental in the manufacture of other hormones, such as dehydroepiandrosterone (DHEA) and pregnenolone. These are produced in the adrenal glands and modulate many bodily functions, including the stress response.

Finally, cholesterol plays a role in every cell of your body. Each of your cells is surrounded by a protective membrane that keeps cellular mechanisms inside and invaders out. Cholesterol is an important component of this protective membrane.

When doctors talk about cholesterol reduction, then, they are not talking about completely banishing cholesterol from the body, but rather trimming the excess fat (literally) and bringing elevated blood levels down to normal.

New Perspectives on Cholesterol

It is fascinating to glance briefly at how scientific understanding of this now common chemical has evolved. Cholesterol was first discovered by a French chemist named Michel Eugène Chevreul in 1815. Chevreul was studying human gallstones and discovered that what we call cholesterol is actually a significant component of these troublesome invaders of the gallbladder and bile ducts. He called his discovery *cholestrine,* from the Latin roots *chole,* meaning "bile," and *stereos,* meaning "solid." The chemical formula for cholesterol was published in 1888, and by 1900, scientists had begun uncovering its molecular structure.

During the decades that followed, cholesterol began to emerge as an increasingly important focus of scientific study. Epidemiologists were noticing that more and more Americans were dying of heart disease. After World War II ended and the government formed the National Institutes of Health to improve all areas of health in the American population, a separate institute called the American Heart Institute was created specifically to study heart disease and disseminate information about it. An increasing number of scientists were devoting time and attention to understanding this insidious and pervasive killer, and cholesterol continued to emerge as the major culprit.

Several major groundbreaking studies confirmed the growing conviction of scientists that cholesterol was implicated in heart disease. The first was conducted in Framingham, Massachusetts, beginning in 1948, and is commonly referred to as the Framingham Study. It measured cholesterol levels in a large group of people (2,282 men and 2,845 women), then followed them for fourteen years to see who would be most likely to develop coronary disease. The results were clear: The higher a person's cholesterol level at the outset of the study, the greater the chance that he or she would develop symptoms of heart disease. People with a total cholesterol of 300 or more milligrams per deciliter (mg/dL) of blood had symptoms more than twice as often as those with a total cholesterol of 150 mg/dL.

A second major study, called the Multiple Risk Factor Intervention Trial (MRFIT), looked at cholesterol levels in 360,000 men. The results were powerful and unequivocal. Participants with total cholesterol levels above 300 mg/dL had a likelihood of dying from CVD that was four times higher than those whose levels were below 180 mg/dL!

As scientific study progressed further, new discoveries were made about cholesterol and heart disease. For example, it was found that the cholesterol level, once though to be a single measurement, was actually composed of several different types of cholesterol. Scientists also began examining other substances in the blood for their association with heart disease.

It appears as though the newfound scientific information that was disseminated to the public had some important impact on the consciousness and lifestyle of Americans. The incidence of heart disease decreased significantly during the years following 1950, when the National Institutes of Health were established. However, the statistics remained disturbingly high. Current estimates point to a staggering 65 million Americans who suffer from high cholesterol, and, if anything, the number has risen over the years. The public health implications of this epidemic of elevated cholesterol were so formidable that in 1985, the National Institutes of Health established the National Cholesterol Education Program (NCEP). This panel of experts issued its first set of guidelines in 1988. The guidelines established clear goals for people with abnormalities in their blood lipids. They were revised in 1993, and then again in 2001, when the third panel expanded them. The new guidelines broadened the focus from cholesterol to the other risk factors, known collectively as syndrome X. (See the National Cholesterol Education Program–Adult Treatment Panel III [NCEP-ATP III] Guidelines and Innovations below.) These guidelines outline new criteria for regarding several blood components as problematic, including the two kinds of cholesterol: HDL and LDL. They also address other risk factors and treatment approaches, which we will be discussing in subsequent chapters.

NCEP-ATP III GUIDELINES AND INNOVATIONS

The following points summarize the recommendations of the National Cholesterol Education Program–Adult Treatment Panel III (NCEP-ATP III):

- They focus on multiple risk factors for the development of cardiovascular disease, not only cholesterol. These include identifying syndrome X, or metabolic syndrome, and elevating diabetes to the status of an independent risk factor.
- They modify the thresholds at which levels of LDL and HDL cholesterol are regarded as problematic. Now, an LDL level of 100 mg/dL or above is considered elevated, and an HDL level of 40 mg/dL or below is considered too low.
- They lower the threshold at which triglycerides are considered elevated to under 200 mg/dL, and recommend treatment for those whose levels are 200 mg/dL or above.
- They recommend a complete blood lipid profile (which measures total cholesterol, LDL, HDL, and triglycerides), not just total cholesterol and HDL, as routine initial screening.
- They encourage therapeutic lifestyle changes (TLC) as the first-line approach for people with few risk factors. These include increased fiber intake, weight loss, and exercise. For people considered to be at high risk, they recommend treatment with LDL-cholesterol–lowering drugs.

HDL and LDL Cholesterol

Years ago, doctors looked at the overall cholesterol level. If it was too high, patients were instructed to bring it down. Today we understand that there are actually two main types of cholesterol: high-density lipoprotein (HDL), which is often called "good" cholesterol, and low-density lipoprotein (LDL), often called "bad" cholesterol. What makes one good and the other bad?

We must begin by understanding how fat moves through your body. If you have ever tried to remove a grease stain from your clothing or scrub a plate on which someone has eaten French fries, you have discovered that fat is not water-soluble. Since blood is water-based, the fats in your body therefore cannot be dissolved in blood for the purpose of transportation. Rather, your body transports fats through the bloodstream by means of a series of proteins that serve as carriers. These protein packages are called *apoproteins*. When a lipid combines with an apoprotein to hitch a ride through your bloodstream, the combination is called a *lipoprotein*.

HDL and LDL cholesterol are lipoproteins. HDL is called *high-density* because it has a much higher ratio of protein to cholesterol than does LDL, or *low-density* (50 percent protein versus 25 percent protein, respectively).

HDL and LDL perform very different functions in the body. The job of HDL is to carry cholesterol to the liver for processing. This ensures that the cholesterol cannot sit around and start accumulating and doing damage in your bloodstream. Instead, the cholesterol is shipped off to the liver. Your liver then proceeds to break it down into substances that can be excreted by the body.

LDL performs an entirely different task. Its job is to transport cholesterol to sites throughout the body. It deposits the cholesterol at the doorstep of damaged cell membranes, where the cholesterol can repair the damage. It deposits the cholesterol at appropriate locations for the building of your sex hormones and the insulation of your nerves. But because the job of LDL is to deposit cholesterol in cells and tissues, it tends to drop bits of cholesterol along the way during the course of its travels. Imagine a truck laden with fruit to be delivered to a series of supermarkets. From time to time, the overloaded truck drops pieces of fruit as it covers thousands of miles of highway.

A good healthy balance means that there isn't so much cholesterol as to overwhelm the LDL system and cause excessive "dropping" of cholesterol in the bloodstream, which can lead to the formation of the plaque that plays such an important and insidious role in the inflammatory process we discussed earlier. Good balance also means that there is plenty of HDL to carry away the fallen "fruit," like the street cleaner trucks that whisk away the garbage on the side of the road. This means that the normal residue of cholesterol left during the travels of LDL to its various destinations will be promptly and efficiently mopped up by HDL.

Now you can understand why HDL is called "good" cholesterol and LDL is called "bad" cholesterol. The more LDL that is present in your blood, the more plaque you will have—especially when the LDL oxidizes and becomes modified as part of the destructive process discussed in chapter 1. The more HDL that is present, the more cleanup of plaque will take place.

The New Guidelines in Practice: Measuring Cholesterol Levels

Up-to-date doctors now test people's cholesterol more frequently, and starting at younger ages. It is recommended that you obtain a regular lipid profile every five years, beginning at age twenty. Once you are over the age of thirty, you should have your levels checked annually, and even more frequently if you have risk factors such as smoking, diabetes, or obesity. Inflammatory lesions can rupture even in relatively young people, and heart disease isn't a condition that affects only older adults.

Make sure that you have been fasting for at least eight hours when you get your blood drawn. If, however, you have been tested on a day when you have already eaten, and your total cholesterol level is higher than 200 mg/dL, or your HDL level is lower than 40 mg/dL, be sure to return when you are fasting to be retested.

What Do the Numbers Mean?

When you have a blood lipid profile done, you will receive several numerical findings on your lab result printout:

- Total cholesterol
- LDL cholesterol
- HDL cholesterol
- Total cholesterol/HDL ratio or LDL/HDL ratio

Although the total cholesterol count is useful, the breakdown of the components is more important. This will show you the levels of "good" and "bad" cholesterol you have, and whether they are in correct balance.

An important note about the ratio: There are two different ratios that laboratories and doctors use—either total cholesterol to HDL cholesterol, or LDL to HDL. Either way, you want this number to be *smaller* rather than bigger! The ratio is expressed in the number of parts total cholesterol or LDL cholesterol over one part HDL cholesterol. The higher the HDL, the greater percentage of blood volume it takes up, and the smaller the number you receive. Table 2.1 lists levels of the various cholesterol readings and ratios and what they mean in terms of cardiovascular risk. I should add that laboratories do not report the numbers in the last two categories as ratios but rather as decimals, which is what you will see on your lab reports. I, however, have given them as ratios to make them easier to understand.

Table 2.1
Cholesterol Levels and Ratios and What They Mean

LDL CHOLESTEROL (mg/dL)	
Level	Category
Under 100	Optimal
100–129	Near or above optimal
130–159	Borderline high
160–189	High
190 or above	Very high

(continued)

Cholesterol Levels and Ratios and What They Mean

TOTAL CHOLESTEROL (mg/dL)

Level	Category
Under 200	Desirable
200–239	Borderline high
240 or above	High

HDL CHOLESTEROL (mg/dL)

Level	Category
Under 40	Low
41–60	Normal
61 or above	High (favorable)

TOTAL CHOLESTEROL : HDL CHOLESTEROL RATIO

Men	Women	Risk Level
3.4 : 1	3.3 : 1	Half the average risk
5 : 1	4.4 : 1	Average risk
9.6 : 1	7.1 : 1	Twice the average risk
23.4 : 1	11 : 1	Three times the average risk

LDL CHOLESTEROL : HDL CHOLESTEROL RATIO

Men	Women	Risk Level
1 : 1	1.5 : 1	Half the average risk
3.6 : 1	3.2 : 1	Average risk
6.3 : 1	5.0 : 1	Twice the average risk
8 : 1	6.1 : 1	Three times the average risk

As you saw in NCEP-ATP III Guidelines and Innovations, physicians are now advised not to regard cholesterol in a vacuum but to see it as part of a constellation of risk factors, including age, triglyceride levels, blood pressure, blood-sugar levels, family history, gender, and weight. The coming chapters will look at all these as well as other risk factors not mentioned in the NCEP-ATP III guidelines.

Putting Cholesterol in Perspective

Although cholesterol is emerging as a more complex subject than originally thought, and although its role has taken on a different perspective, this does not mean you can disregard having elevated cholesterol levels if you have been so diagnosed. Remember that cholesterol is ultimately the most important building block of plaque. Normal cholesterol levels do not necessarily guarantee that you will be free of cardiovascular disease, but high cholesterol levels mean that you are *definitely* at high risk. It is imperative that you take this risk seriously and use natural methods to lower your cholesterol levels, even if you have no other risk factors.

I stress *natural* methods because while the NCEP-ATP III guidelines might pay lip service to the role of TLC for reducing LDL cholesterol, in reality the reflexive focus is on cholesterol-lowering drugs. This is especially the case for people who have more than one risk factor. While I accept the need for aggressive action, I believe that the thorough holistic approach of the DEAR program *is* aggressive and has fewer side effects than drug therapy.

A Look at Medications

What types of medications are being prescribed? What's right with them, and what's wrong with them?

Most cholesterol-lowering prescription medications belong to a class of pharmaceuticals called *statin drugs*. Although a second class of cholesterol reduction agents called *fibrates* exists, these are not as powerful or as effective as the statins, and they are less frequently prescribed. There is also another class of medications, *bile acid sequestrants,* that can be used for high cholesterol. Let us look at each of these in turn.

STATIN DRUGS

Statins are designed to block the manufacture of cholesterol in the liver by inhibiting the function of the enzyme *HMG-CoA reductase*, a necessary player in the chain of events that leads to cholesterol synthesis. Some statin drugs also increase the number of hepatic LDL receptors, the receptors within liver cells that are responsible for "grabbing" LDL ("bad") cholesterol particles and breaking them down. So the drug functions to reduce the amount of cholesterol being synthesized and to break down some of the cholesterol that has already been synthesized before it can be released into the bloodstream.

But there is a big downside to statins.

HMG-CoA reductase also has a protective effect on muscle tissue. Without the protection of this enzyme, muscle cells begin to break down. Left unchecked, the waste products of the muscular breakdown begin to accumulate in the kidneys, literally flooding and overwhelming them until they shut down. A similar mechanism may be involved with nerves and brain cells that require cholesterol for regular upkeep. Without the action of this enzyme, these cells suffer. This may cause side effects such as memory loss, difficulty concentrating, irritability, anxiety, and depression.

Nerves in other parts of the body, not only the brain, can be affected by these medications. A Danish study published in the journal *Neurology* reported that statin drugs could increase the risk of developing peripheral neuropathy—damage to the peripheral nerves that causes weakness, numbness, tingling, and pain in the hands and feet.

But most people who take statins and begin developing muscle aches or memory lapses do not associate these symptoms with their medication. Although young people with elevated cholesterol are usually given prescriptions for statins, the preponderance of individuals who take these medications are older adults. When a woman in her fifties or sixties complains to the doctor about aches and pains or being forgetful, the most common response is "you're menopausal" or "you're having a senior moment." Men are treated to a similar response: "It's a normal part of aging." These responses are typical, even when the person is complaining of serious impairment due to an undetected burgeoning illness. Certainly, more subtle complaints are all too easily dismissed and people are often reluctant to report them, erroneously believing that they are being hypochondriacs. I'm here to tell you that growing older does *not* necessarily entail feeling stiff and achy, being edgy and irritable, or having memory lapses. The effects of all medications, not only statins, cannot be ignored.

Although many doctors dismiss these side effects, an increasing number of patients are becoming concerned and are associating their disturbing symptoms with their use of statin drugs. Many people stop taking their medications because of concerns about side effects. In fact, according to Dr. William Roberts, editor in chief of the prestigious *American Journal of Cardiology,* about half of people who are put on lipid-lowering drugs stop using the medication within one year, and only 25 percent continue treatment for two years.

Many of my colleagues have confirmed that their patients often discard their statin drugs because of unpleasant side effects. This pattern is apparent in my own medical practice, where I am regularly consulted by patients seeking alternatives to the statin drugs prescribed by a primary-care physician or cardiologist. The negative publicity surrounding this category of medication following the recall of the popular drug cerivastatin (Baycol) validated their fears and raised concerns in those who had not previously been worried. In August of 2001, this statin drug was taken off the shelves after it was linked with more than 52 deaths caused by the drug's serious side effects related to muscle wasting and the development of a potentially lethal condition known as rhabdomyolysis. Needless to say, this caused great public concern worldwide to the more than six million users of this drug who were now forced to seek an alternative. Lawsuits were filed against Bayer, the manufacturer, and the first

> **STATIN PRECAUTIONS AND WARNING SIGNS**
>
> If you must take a statin drug, you should be aware of the following precautions to help you take it as safely as possible and warning signs that may signal developing problems:
>
> - Inform your doctor about all other medications and herbs you are taking. Do not take both a statin and a fibrate or blood thinner.
> - Avoid drinking grapefruit juice. Some studies have suggested that it can interact negatively with statin drugs.
> - Discontinue use of the statin and seek alternatives immediately if you experience any of the following:
>   - muscle pain or weakness
>   - brown urine
>   - numbness, pain, or tingling in your extremities
>   - memory or concentration problems
>   - unusual fatigue
>   - impotence
> - Make sure your doctor performs regular tests of liver function and muscle enzymes. While these tests are not perfect—there are a significant number of reports of people experiencing the above symptoms whose test results are normal—they are at least a step in the right direction.

was settled in September 2002. What is disturbing is that the other statin drugs utilize the same mechanism of action within the body and carry similar risks. Since then, the number of patients seeking alternatives has increased dramatically, and their concerns are completely justified.

Aren't You Being an Alarmist?

Proponents of statin drugs have defended their use by noting that cerivastatin was markedly different from other statins in potency—it was effective at very low dosages. They theorize that the alarming reactions to cerivastatin were caused by overdosing on the drug and that the lower doses used by the other agents confer protection on users.

They also note that most of the deaths from cerivastatin were suffered by individuals using the medication in conjunction with other therapies—particularly another cholesterol-lowering medication, gemfibrozil (Lopid). Other drugs that have been associated with side effects when taken in combination with statins are certain blood thinners, antifungal medications, and some antibiotics.

My own opinion is that being concerned about side effects of statin drugs is not being alarmist, but being responsible. There are many wonderful, equally effective, and far safer natural alternatives to these agents for cholesterol reduction and these should be used as first-line approaches, with statin drugs being used only as a last resort if natural means fail. This gives the body a chance to strengthen and heal itself and protects the liver and muscles from the potential adverse effects of statins.

It's especially frustrating that some studies have implied that statin drugs should not be taken together with antioxidants. Considering what we know about the inflammatory process and the essential part that antioxidants can play in rectifying it, a medication that curtails or precludes the use of antioxidants is at best misguided. At worst, it is downright counterproductive.

The same line of reasoning applies to the depletion of an important substance in the body called *coenzyme Q_{10},* which is instrumental in stabilizing the cardiac membranes responsible for the heart's electrical conduction system, thereby preventing or rectifying arrhythmias. Coenzyme Q_{10} deficiency is associated with congestive heart failure, angina, high blood pressure, and poor exercise tolerance. (You will learn more about this amazing agent in chapter 12.) Again, any medication that depletes such an important part of the body's natural ability to maintain cardiac health should be avoided. Co Q_{10} depletion can also contribute to some of the aches, pains, and fatigue I have seen in so many people who take statin drugs. In fact, some drug companies are considering adding coenzyme Q_{10} to their statin patent to offset this problem.

Finally, a few recent studies are beginning to question at least some of the claims boasted by the proponents of statin drugs—specifically, an international study conducted by researchers in thirty-seven countries in 2002. They observed 12,365 subjects who had experienced acute coronary syndromes during the previous three to four months. These conditions included heart attacks and unstable angina, as well as several other conditions. The purpose of the study was to evaluate the effectiveness of initiating treatment with statins soon (less than seven days) after the coronary event. The study found that statin drugs did not improve the outcomes of those patients who were treated. I believe that additional studies may also begin to call into question the praise that statins have received in the medical community and will support the use of natural alternatives to these agents.

Needless to say, a natural, statin-free program will involve more effort and lifestyle changes than a protocol that demands little more than reaching for a pill bottle. In fact, according to physician and author Dean Ornish, M.D., this is the reason for the increase in statin drug prescriptions—even the NCEP-ATP III do not go far enough with recommendations for lifestyle changes to assure dramatic cholesterol reduction, so medication is needed.

Perhaps the reason for the NCEP's modest guidelines is an awareness of the American mentality. Lifestyle alterations are difficult and require not only profound commitment to one's health but a willingness to examine broader issues, such as the time and effort involved in reaching a goal. We Americans are a speed-oriented society. We need only turn on the television sets to realize that speed is the most valued commodity in any product or service—how fast the pizza is delivered, how fast the painkiller works, how fast the modem connects. Our ancestors had to wait for crops to grow, but we need only to visit the supermarket and take the bread or vegetable off the shelves. Our grandparents sent letters and, in dire emergencies, telegrams; we have faxes and e-mails that work instantaneously and without even the effort of walking to the post office or corner mailbox. We have come to expect the same rapid, magic-bullet solutions to our health problems. Alas, our bodies were not constructed to function that way. The DEAR program, which requires dietary changes, nutritional supplementation, exercise, and stress reduction may take longer and involve some inconvenience, but it will ultimately pay off in the long term with safer, more effective cholesterol reduction and good health.

FIBRATES

Fibrates are fat-regulating agents that exercise a modest LDL-cholesterol–lowering effect in some people. However, they actually can raise LDL levels in other people, so they are prescribed with caution. Their real strength lies in decreasing levels of triglycerides—a category of blood fat—and very low-density lipoprotein (VLDL), which transports triglycerides through the bloodstream as a package, stimulating excess insulin production and wreaking all sorts of other damage. An agent that lowers these can reduce a person's vulnerability to insulin resistance, type 2 diabetes, and cardiovascular disease. (The connections among all of these conditions will be examined in detail in chapter 5.) The mechanism of action has not been firmly established; however, it appears that fibrates inhibit the decomposition of fat and decrease the extraction of free fatty acids in the liver. This reduces the ability of the liver to manufacture and secrete triglycerides. Additionally, fibrates inhibit the synthesis of a substance called *apolipoprotein B,* which carries the VLDL that, in turn, binds to and carries triglycerides throughout the body. Fibrates may help lower LDL cholesterol by accelerating the turnover and removal of cholesterol from the liver and increasing its excretion from the body.

Some people report experiencing gastrointestinal discomfort from fibrates, while others experience dizziness and fatigue. Muscle aches and pains have also been associated with fibrates—perhaps for a similar reason that statin drugs cause these symptoms. The inhibition of cholesterol production robs muscles of cholesterol needed to repair and build muscle cells.

Fibrates and statins do not mix well together. In fact, one of the individuals who died of rhabdomyolysis (a serious disease characterized by muscle breakdown causing kidney failure) was taking Baycol together with Lopid. Make sure you do not use these drugs together!

BILE ACID SEQUESTRANTS

Cholestyramine and colestipol, the most common of these agents, are actually ammonium salts. They bind to bile acids in the intestines, thereby promoting their excretion. This puts more cholesterol to work creating new bile acids, resulting in decreased levels of blood cholesterol. Bile acid sequestrants have occasionally increased triglyceride levels. Even more serious, they can disrupt absorption of vitamins such as vitamins A, D, E, and K, which are fat-soluble and essential for many bodily functions.

A NEW CLASS OF MEDICATIONS

In October 2002, a new medication called epetimibe (Zetia) was approved for cholesterol reduction. It is the first in a class of medications not yet formally named, and simply called *add-on* because it is designed to complement and potentiate the effects of statin drugs for people who do not achieve a sufficient reduction in LDL cholesterol levels with statins alone. Epetimibe works by inhibiting cholesterol absorption in the intestine. Because this medication is so new, it is too soon to know whether any unexpected adverse effects may occur once the medication is popularized. As of now, it has not been associated with muscle aches or rhabdomyolysis when used as a self-standing therapy (in other words, independent of statin drugs).

WHEN IS DRUG THERAPY INDICATED?

Many of my patients have turned to me, a holistic practitioner, as a last resort. My holistically oriented colleagues report that the same is true for most of their patients, who regard "alternative medicine" as something to try when conventional medicine has failed. (Of course, by the time a person has reached the end of the conventional road, it is sometimes too late for alternative medicine to be effective.) My philosophy is exactly reverse. I believe that conventional medicine should be used if holistic approaches have not proved effective. I occasionally prescribe statin drugs as a short-term emergency measure while the real work of the DEAR program is underway, or as a last resort if the gentler holistic measures are not successful.

When I do prescribe drugs, I begin with much smaller doses than those generally prescribed. In fact, some research has suggested that many of the negative side effects associated with medications can be due to overdosing. A study conducted at Georgetown University examined the recommended doses of 354 prescription drugs released from 1980 to 1999. In 73 of these drugs (21 percent), the instructions on the label had to be altered after the drug came on the market. Most of these corrections consisted of a reduction in the original dose or a new restriction for certain groups of people, such as those with liver or kidney disease.

According to Jay Cohen, M.D., of the Departments of Family and Preventive Medicine and Psychiatry at the University of California in San Diego, "rational dosing" is key for successful use of statins, not only for achieving target LDL cholesterol levels but also for avoiding adverse effects. In fact, each doubling of the statin dosage also doubles the incidence of excessive liver enzyme elevations. He cites a study that found 52 percent of patients achieved LDL cholesterol reductions with just 0.2 mg/day of cerivastatin—half the manufacturer's recommended initial dosage.

So if you must take medication, ask your doctor to start you out on a tiny dose—perhaps a fraction of the manufacturer-recommended dosage, while you simultaneously implement the DEAR program. It is likely that this will be sufficient to address your immediate situation while the long-term work is being accomplished.

 Additional Clues in the Blood

... That nothing do but meditate on blood ...
—William Shakespeare

I'm sure it came as no surprise when you read in chapter 2 that elevated cholesterol levels are one of the leading causes of cardiovascular disease. You may be surprised to learn how many other equally important culprits have been discovered by today's scientists. Since about one-quarter of all people who develop CVD do not smoke, are not obese, do not have high blood pressure, and have normal cholesterol levels, investigators have long sought other clues to identify a risk of CVD before symptoms appear. New markers have emerged, even as the atherosclerotic process has been reframed and refined from the simple mechanistic model of clogged plumbing to the more complex, dynamic model of inflammation that we discussed in chapter 1. These include triglycerides, which have been known for a long time but whose significance is becoming clearer as the pieces of the syndrome X puzzle are being assembled. Other more recently identified markers include elevated blood levels of homocysteine, C-reactive protein, fibrinogen, and lipoprotein (a).

Elevated Triglycerides

Like cholesterol, triglycerides are necessary in small quantities. They can be manufactured in the liver or absorbed from the food you eat. Triglycerides are either used by the body as a source of energy or stored as fat. Like cholesterol, triglycerides are not water-soluble, so if they must be moved from point A to point B by your blood (which is, after all, your body's transport system), they must be attached or packaged properly for transportation. Like cholesterol, they must be carried by apoproteins. The new combined entity, the lipoprotein, that transports most of your triglycerides is called very low-density lipoprotein, or VLDL (not to be confused with LDL cholesterol). It consists primarily of triglycerides, together with an additional protein and a small quantity of cholesterol.

Numerous studies have determined that people with elevated triglycerides have a higher risk of CVD than people with normal triglyceride levels, and the NCEP-ATP III guidelines have included high triglycerides as a risk factor for CVD.

Table 3.1 summarizes the new NCEP-ATP III guidelines for triglycerides.

TABLE 3.1
NCEP-ATP III Guidelines for Triglycerides

Level	Category
Under 150 mg/dL	Normal
150–199 mg/dL	Borderline high
200–400 mg/dL	High
500 mg/dL or higher	Very high

According to the new guidelines, the first-line treatment approach for elevated triglycerides is to intensify weight management and increase physical activity and to reduce consumption of sugars. Additionally, it is assumed that by reducing levels of LDL cholesterol (which often, though not always, goes hand in hand with elevated triglycerides) and raising levels of HDL cholesterol, triglyceride levels also will be normalized. This may or may not work, which is why I recommend additional supplementation.

Elevated Homocysteine

In 1969, a pathologist named Kilmer McCully, M.D., suggested that cholesterol was not the only culprit in the development of atherosclerosis. He developed this theory after autopsies on young children with a rare genetic disease called *homocysteinuria* revealed the presence of atherosclerotic plaque. These children all had abnormally high levels of homocysteine, a by-product of protein metabolism found in the blood. He began to wonder if homocysteine could be implicated in atherosclerosis of healthy people as well. His theory was so threatening to the conventional model of heart disease that he was actually asked to leave Harvard Medical School. Now, a little over three decades later, Dr. McCully's research has been vindicated by numerous studies, and homocysteine is accepted as a major risk factor for the development of cardiovascular disease.

Current research suggests that as many as 42 percent of strokes, 30 percent of cases of CVD, and 28 percent of cases of peripheral vascular disease might be caused by high levels of homocysteine. It is possible that as many as half of those with congenital hyperhomocysteinemia (elevated blood homocysteine) experience a heart- or brain-related event involving a blood clot before age thirty. Of these people, 20 percent do not survive.

A landmark meta-analysis (a study that combines results of many other studies) found that each 5 micromole per liter (μmol/L) rise in fasting homocysteine levels increased the risk of coronary heart disease by 1.6 times in men and 1.8 times in women—a finding comparable to the extra risk conferred by other more "traditional" lipid factors, such as cholesterol and triglycerides. Other studies confirm this astounding finding, which has also been borne out in my clinical experience.

What is homocysteine, and what is its connection to cardiovascular disease?

Homocysteine is generated by the normal breakdown of an amino acid called *methionine*. *Amino acids* are the building blocks of proteins, which are indispensable ingredients of a healthy diet. Proteins are integral to the healthy functioning of our bodies—especially important for muscle building and production of brain chemicals called *neurotransmitters* that transmit signals and information between nerve cells in our brains. Some of these amino acids are called *essential*. Although they are essential in the traditional sense—we can't manage without them—the term *essential,* as used here, is a is a technical word meaning that our own bodies cannot manufacture them. Certain amino acids must be imported into our bodies by means of our diets. There are nine essential amino acids we must take in when we eat. If we have adequate quantities of these and metabolize them effectively, we have the raw materials our bodies need to manufacture all the other proteins necessary for good health and functioning. Methionine is one of the nine essential amino acids.

Homocysteine is generated during the metabolism of methionine. It is a normal by-product of this process and performs two functions. It is part of a chain of reactions that produces several more proteins. First it's transformed into *cystathionine.* This product, in turn, is used to manufacture *cysteine,* a non-essential amino acid. Once cysteine has done its job, it is broken down by the body and excreted in the urine. A second function of homocysteine involves a complicated series of events that ultimately generates more methionine in the body.

Like cholesterol, homocysteine isn't bad. It's essential (literally) to our health and survival. The problem arises when homocysteine levels are too high, either due to an inherited predisposition or because the chemicals that the body needs to enact all these complicated processes are missing. This takes place especially at the point at which homocysteine is being broken down for excretion. When certain vitamins, enzymes, and nutrients called *cofactors* are missing, the homocysteine cannot be adequately broken down, and so it builds up in the body.

Elevated homocysteine is toxic to the endothelium. For starters, it promotes free-radical formation and is hostile to the membranes of many cellular surfaces, including that of the arterial endothelium.

Plus, excessive homocysteine promotes clotting, both within the bloodstream and along the endothelium. Blood clots can be fatal, as you know, because they can cause blockages in blood vessels, especially those leading to the heart or brain. And the presence of extra clotting factors worsens the process of plaque formation.

Elevated homocysteine can undo even the best-intentioned medical and surgical intervention for CVD. Addressing this imbalance has been shown to increase the success rates of treatment. For example, researchers discovered that homocysteine-lowering therapy (consisting of taking a combination of vitamins B_6, B_{12}, and folic acid) significantly reduced the incidence of restenosis (re-narrowing) of the arteries in patients who had undergone angioplasty, or the "balloon" procedure, to open clogged arteries. These patients were treated for six months, then evaluated after another six months. Patients who had received this treatment remained freer of heart attack, plaque, and restenosis even six months after they had discontinued treatment, suggesting that the positive outcomes are not just temporary. (In my opinion, however, treatment should be continued because it is extremely safe and inexpensive.)

Although the role of homocysteine in CVD is increasingly being accepted in the medical community, many cardiologists are still not aware of it or are reluctant to incorporate it into their testing and treatment protocols.

There is an array of reasons why a person might experience elevated levels of homocysteine. These include the following:

- Chronic illness, such as cancer, psoriasis, kidney dysfunction, systemic lupus erythematosus, and others
- Enzyme deficiencies
- Increasing age

- Male gender
- The use of certain medications, including carbamezapine (Tegretol), colestipol (Colestid), methotrexate (Rheumatrex), nicotinic acid (Niacor, Niaspan), phenytoin (Dilantin), and thiazide-based diuretics
- Solid organ transplantation
- Smoking
- Vitamin deficiencies, particularly deficiencies of folic acid (folate), vitamin B_6, and vitamin B_{12}

If you are affected by any of these conditions, you need to be especially vigilant of your homocysteine levels because you are at increased risk for the development of CVD. Finally, you should be aware that if you have had blood drawn during an acute illness—the flu, for example, or some other infection by a virus or bacteria—your homocysteine levels are likely to be elevated. This is a normal systemic response to illness. In such a case, it is advisable to have your blood retested when your illness has subsided.

Although laboratory testing for homocysteine is available, the American Heart Association (AHA) has so far recommended routine testing only for certain people:

- Individuals with atherosclerosis, even in the absence of other risk factors
- Individuals with premature atherosclerosis (younger than age sixty)
- Individuals at risk for premature atherosclerosis, including people with a family history of atherosclerosis, smokers, and people with high blood pressure
- People with chronic illnesses (see above)
- Individuals who have had a venous thrombosis (blood clot in the vein)

I believe that we do not need to wait for the blessing of the AHA to order this inexpensive and potentially life-saving test for everyone. During the past ten years, I have found that at least 25 percent of my cardiac patients have homocysteine levels that put them at risk. If I did not routinely check homocysteine, this important factor would be overlooked and these patients would not receive appropriate therapy. If you fall into any of the categories recognized by the AHA as recommended for testing, it is *essential* for you to make sure your doctor orders this test. Table 3.2 indicates evaluations of different ranges for homocysteine.

Table 3.2
Homocysteine Levels and What They Mean

Level	Category
Under 10µmol/L	Normal
10.1–15 µmol/L	Borderline high
15.1–20 µol/L	High
Over 20 µol/L	Very high

Elevated C-Reactive Protein

Manufactured in the liver in response to tissue inflammation and infection, *C-reactive protein* (CRP) has long been recognized as a marker of inflammation in conditions such as rheumatoid arthritis, vasculitis, and infectious diseases. But its usefulness as a clue to the presence of an inflammatory process that can be related to cardiovascular disease is relatively new. About two decades ago, two British scientists suggested that CRP was an important marker of certain injuries to cardiac tissue. But the early tests were too crude to be much use in fine-tuning the relationship between CRP and cardiac disease.

As scientists continued to piece together the vast and often confusing puzzle of cardiovascular disease, and as the role of inflammation continued to emerge as critical to the process, they refined the testing for

CRP. By the early 1990s, they had developed a more standardized test for CRP that could reliably predict cardiac risk. This test, known as the *high-sensitivity CRP (hs-CRP)*, also called *cardiac CRP*, assay became valuable in assessing the degree of inflammation in the blood vessels that could lead to dangerously unstable plaques. Nowadays, most labs perform the hs-CRP test routinely, and the results of the major studies of CRP no longer make special mention of hs-CRP because the newest assays are sufficiently sensitive to detect CRP without being specially noted. However, I still request that my lab perform the *cardiac* CRP test to be on the safe side, and you can ask your doctor to do the same.

Table 3.3 summarizes the ranges of CRP that I have found most useful.

TABLE 3.3
C-Reactive Protein Levels and What They Mean

Level	Category
1 mg/L or under	Normal
1.01–1.5 mg/L	Borderline high
1.6–2.0 mg/L	High
2.01 mg/L and over	Very high

What might raise CRP levels? The jury is still out concerning the exact role that elevated CRP might play in the atherosclerotic inflammatory process. Certain factors appear to increase its presence in the blood, including:

- Smoking
- Diabetes
- Estrogen supplementation
- Obesity
- Lack of exercise/sedentary lifestyle
- Infections

Although CRP testing is most commonly recommended for middle-aged and older men and women (and postmenopausal women of all ages), I recommend it for all my patients. According to some reports, it can predict heart attacks and strokes up to six years before they occur, and even individuals with slightly elevated blood levels appear to be at higher risk for CVD and its complications, regardless of age, gender, general health, or the presence of other risk factors. So as far as I'm concerned, this test is too important to pass up.

There are a few important caveats to note here:

- When you go to your doctor, make sure you ask for the hs-CRP or cardiac CRP test. While most labs now routinely perform this specialized test, a few do not, so it is worth making sure that you are receiving the correct test.
- Some labs report the results in milligrams per deciliter (mg/dL), while others use milligrams per liter (mg/L)—which yields a tenfold difference in results! Pay attention to which system your laboratory uses so that you can understand them correctly. If you aren't sure, ask your doctor.
- If you have an infection in your system—bronchitis or a urinary tract infection, for example—you can have elevated levels of CRP. So avoid having your blood drawn if you are ill. And if your results show an abnormality that you question or that seems inconsistent with your lifestyle, make sure to repeat them—perhaps you were suffering from an undetected infection when you were tested.

Elevated Fibrinogen

Fibrinogen is a blood protein essential for proper clotting. Too much fibrinogen, however, can cause excessive clotting in the blood and has been implicated in the formation of atherosclerotic plaque lesions. And like CRP, elevated fibrinogen is believed to be a signal of vascular inflammation.

Studies have linked high levels of fibrinogen to increased risk of CVD. For example, the Physicians' Health Study II, an ongoing randomized trial that began in 1997, found that apparently healthy men with an excessive concentration of fibrinogen (343 mg/dL or higher) had approximately twice the risk of having a heart attack as those with lower fibrinogen levels. Another study of 2,709 apparently healthy and symptom-free Native Americans enrolled in the Strong Heart Study found that the third of the group with high fibrinogen levels were more likely than the two-thirds with lower levels to have at least one preclinical abnormality, such as arterial stiffness, or dysfunction of the myocardium of the heart. The investigators suggested that elevated fibrinogen might be a marker of subclinical atherosclerosis, endothelial dysfunction, and other forms of vascular disease.

This is especially significant because of the subtlety and sensitivity of this test. If it is predicting "preclinical atherosclerosis," this means that it can enable physicians to nip the process in the bud, at the very beginning, before major inflammation and other symptoms set in. This can be an extremely useful preventive tool.

If a patient's lab results show elevated levels of fibrinogen, I immediately recommend the CARE diet (which you will learn about in part 2), with specific emphasis on olive oil, fish such as salmon (which is rich in EPA, an essential fatty acid that is known to act as a blood thinner), and foods such as garlic, onions, and shallots that are high in allium, a blood-thinning nutrient. As long as you don't have a history of alcoholism, I suggest taking an occasional glass of red wine, which has been associated with a decrease in fibrinogen levels. Depending on a patient's other risk factors, I create a supplement program, with special emphasis on vitamins C and E. In particular, vitamin E has blood-thinning effects.

Elevated Lipoprotein (a)

Elevated *lipoprotein (a)*—abbreviated as *Lp(a)*—is a serious risk factor in the development of CVD. It is a deadly component of LDL cholesterol and, like fibrinogen, appears to play an important role in clot formation and the inhibition of blood thinning. One study found that individuals with high blood levels of Lp(a) were 70 percent more likely to have a heart attack than those with lower levels. Lp(a) has been found to be highly correlated with the risk of restenosis after balloon angioplasty. In fact, of all the risk factors, elevated Lp(a) is the one that most closely predicts the redevelopment of blockage in the newly opened artery.

Table 3.4 indicates the normal and abnormal levels of Lp(a).

Table 3.4
Lipoprotein (a) Levels and What They Mean

Level	Category
20 mg/dL or under	Normal
21–30 mg/dL	Borderline high
31–40 mg/dL	High
41 mg/dL and over	Very high

Lp(a) has not yet emerged center stage as a player in the cardiovascular drama. Many physicians either are still not aware of it or do not test for it during checkups.

There appears to be a strong familial tendency toward elevated Lp(a) levels. If parents have this problem, about 50 percent of their children can be expected to develop it as well. Whatever the cause, it can be extremely difficult to lower Lp(a) levels. Diet and exercise alone have yielded disappointing results. I generally recommend aggressive treatment—especially if there are other risk factors, such as elevated homocysteine or fibrinogen. Vitamin C and niacin have been most helpful, although I use other supplements as well.

 High Blood Pressure: The "Silent" Killer

... who make no noise are dangerous.
—Jean de La Fontaine

Most people know that hypertension (high blood pressure) is dangerous. It is now common to see blood pressure–screening stands in shopping malls and community centers, and even on street corners. Many hospitals conduct regular free blood pressure readings as a community service. Obviously, this communicates an important message: Hypertension is dangerous and should be avoided. Hypertension has also become part of our everyday idiom—"Don't upset Mom, you'll give her high blood pressure."

It is my experience, however, that most people do not quite realize how dangerous hypertension can be, or what type of danger it poses. Hypertension is one of the leading risk factors for cardiovascular disease. It affects an estimated 50 million American adults (that's one-quarter of the entire adult population of the United States!). Studies show, however, that only 68 percent of those affected are aware of their condition, and only 27 percent have it under control. Each year, 2 million new cases of hypertension are diagnosed. The risk increases with age: 64 percent of people over age seventy suffer from it. The risk also varies by ethnicity: African-Americans have significantly more risk of developing hypertension than do other segments of the population.

What is insidious about high blood pressure is that it has no symptoms. The reason there are so many undiagnosed people with this condition is that many people don't become aware of it until they have a stroke or heart attack. This is why it's so important to have your blood pressure monitored regularly at annual medical checkups or whenever you visit your doctor for any reason.

What Is Hypertension?

Let's start with a simple definition. *Hypertension* means "high blood pressure." *Hyper* means "high," while *tension* refers to the pressure within the arteries. This pressure is caused by the pumping action of the heart, which pushes blood into and through the arteries. There must be enough pressure for the blood to keep a steady forward motion. This pressure—the amount of tension that pushes against the arterial walls—is determined by *cardiac output* (the quantity of blood pumped out of the heart) and *peripheral resistance* (the general tone of the arteries).

Blood pressure is measured in millimeters of mercury (mm Hg). This does not mean that you have mercury in your bloodstream, thank goodness. It refers to the sphygmomanometer, the instrument that doctors use to measure blood pressure. This is a glass tube, scored with numbers, in which a column of mercury rises and falls until it reaches the appropriate measurement—like an old-fashioned home thermometer.

When your blood pressure is measured, you get two numbers. The top number is your *systolic blood pressure*. This is the highest pressure in your arteries during *systole*—when the heart is contracting. The bottom number is called *diastolic blood pressure*. It is the lowest pressure within your arteries during *diastole,* when your heart is relaxing and refilling with blood.

It may surprise you to learn that your blood pressure does not remain constant throughout the day. Although an average blood pressure is usually around 120/80 mm Hg, blood pressure rises during times of exercise or stress. Sometimes, the anxiety of being in the doctor's office can create internal stress that actually raises blood pressure. This is often called *white-coat hypertension.* Blood pressure also fluctuates depending on whether you are sitting, standing, or moving around. This is why a correct diagnosis requires at least three readings on separate occasions.

High blood pressure is a broad term that encompasses several different conditions of varying severity. For starters, you can have elevated systolic pressure with normal diastolic pressure—or vice versa. Each of these circumstances is associated with a different set of risks. High levels of systolic pressure are associated with a higher risk of CVD, while high levels of diastolic pressure are more likely to cause kidney damage or damage to peripheral blood vessels. Some people have elevations in both.

High blood pressure cannot be lightly dismissed. For each 7.5 mm elevation of diastolic blood pressure, there is a 29-percent increase in the risk of cardiovascular disease. So even a mild elevation can be a sign of trouble, especially because it can (and usually does) progress to higher and more dangerous levels. The same holds true for a moderate elevation. A severe elevation (systolic pressure of 180 to 209 and a diastolic pressure above 90) requires immediate and urgent evaluation and treatment.

How Hypertension Contributes to Cardiovascular Disease

People with uncontrolled high blood pressure are about three times more likely to suffer from coronary artery disease, six times more likely to suffer from congestive heart failure, and seven times more likely to have a stroke than people with normal or controlled blood pressure. Why? Because the heart is forced to work harder than normal to push the blood through the vessels. The extra strain weakens the heart, leading to conditions such as congestive heart failure.

Hypertension causes CVD for another reason. It is no coincidence that about 80 percent of individuals with hypertension also have problematic levels of blood fats (cholesterol and triglycerides), and about half have insulin resistance or diabetes. Hypertension often appears as a component of the constellation of conditions that make up syndrome X, and the fact that they so often occur together provides an important clue to why hypertension is so destructive. Scientists are still assembling the pieces of this complex puzzle, but the emerging picture appears to point to the endothelial wall of the artery as the prime suspect. When you have elevated blood pressure, the delicate endothelial walls are constantly being stressed and stretched by the extra pressure exerted by blood surging through. Although the blood vessels are designed to stretch, they are not designed for this amount of consistent pressure. Think of what happens to the elastic on your clothing if you stretch it too far—it eventually loses its elasticity and becomes "stuck."

The same thing happens to your endothelium. The connective tissue holding the endothelial cells together becomes stretched, leaving larger openings between the cells. Stray molecules of cholesterol and triglycerides have an easier time wriggling between the cells and forming a fatty streak.

Now the connection between these apparently disparate conditions begins to make more sense. The higher the blood pressure, the larger the openings along the endothelial walls, and the more the accumulation of plaque. Circulating triglycerides cannot be properly disposed of, and they add to the debris. The presence of plaque further stiffens the blood vessel walls, which become increasingly dysfunctional. Blood no longer circulates efficiently, which puts even greater strain on the heart. The inefficient blood flow compromises the delivery of oxygen to organs of the body such as the heart, brain, and kidneys. This is one major reason why individuals with hypertension so often suffer heart attacks, strokes, and kidney damage.

Another reason is that the less-efficient blood vessel walls no longer perform their job of serving as a barrier between the blood within the vessels and the "outside" world—the world of organs, connective tissue, bone, muscle, and other bodily equipment. Invaders can cross the barrier, wreaking havoc in the organs and within the blood. The carefully controlled balance that is usually maintained by the endothelium of "good" and "bad" mediators, pro- and anticlotting factors, pro- and anti-inflammatory substances, and pro- and antioxidant chemicals becomes disrupted.

All of this activity takes place while the person goes about his or her daily life, unaware of the war being waged within the bloodstream. As I have mentioned, hypertension is often called the "silent killer" because it can be present without any symptoms at all. However, in some people, it can cause one or more of the following:

- Fatigue
- Headaches
- Confusion
- Changes in vision
- Excessive sweating
- Ruddy complexion

If you are experiencing any of these symptoms for no known reason, you should consult your health-care practitioner immediately. But remember that many people have none of these symptoms until they suffer from a heart attack or stroke, which is why regular checkups are so important.

Hypertension can do its damage directly on the heart itself. Long-standing elevations in blood pressure can cause the left ventricle (the main pump of the heart) to stiffen and enlarge. The entire heart eventually enlarges and becomes less efficient.

Treating Hypertension

Hypertension is the most common reason for visits to physicians' offices in America, and the number-one condition for which drugs are prescribed. The annual expenditure for antihypertensive prescription drugs is over $10 billion per year, and this amount is projected to exceed $25 billion by the year 2007! However, according to the National Health and Nutrition Examination Survey (NHANES) III, only 27 percent of the hypertensive population had controlled their blood pressure to the desired goal—less than 140/90. And although the money spent on antihypertensive medications has doubled since 1990, the percentage of those whose blood pressure is successfully under control has actually declined since then.

These are deeply disturbing figures. It is clear that, despite the best efforts of the drug companies, the central reasons for hypertension are not being addressed. Perhaps this is because medication is not the answer, although it can be a short-term stopgap for some people with an especially serious problem. The real answer to blood-pressure control lies in lifestyle changes. The American Heart Association recommends following a healthy diet, restricting sodium intake, quitting smoking, losing weight if necessary, and moderating alcohol consumption. Regular exercise and stress reduction are essential. These are all components of the DEAR program. If you follow the guidelines in part 2 of this book, you should experience a significant reduction in blood pressure.

5 Diabetes and Cardiovascular Disease: Making the Link

> *... the taste of sweetness, whereof a little*
> *More than a little is by much too much.*
> —WILLIAM SHAKESPEARE

According to recent statistics, diabetes affects over 16 million Americans—a staggering number. It takes a toll on many areas of health, but most people do not associate it with heart disease. Sure, they think of circulatory problems and are acutely aware of the potential danger of an infection in their extremities. In fact, a study of 900 physicians commissioned by the American Diabetes Association and the American College of Cardiology found that 68 percent of people with diabetes were unaware of their increased risk for heart disease and stroke. The same study suggested that many physicians have been remiss in focusing more attention on blood-sugar measures than on fat and blood pressure control. This is quite disturbing, considering that the NCEP-ATP III guidelines have moved diabetes to the status of an independent risk factor for CVD, as important as high cholesterol. This chapter will help you understand why diabetes poses so much danger to the heart.

What Is Diabetes?

Diabetes is a disease caused by the malfunction of the pancreas—a long, thin organ located behind the stomach. The pancreas actually produces many important digestive enzymes, but it is best known for the production of a hormone called *insulin*. Insulin binds to the glucose (sugar) that comes from the breakdown of the food you eat, then transports the glucose to the cells of your liver and muscles, where it is stored for future use as fuel. When your pancreas is functioning normally, your blood-sugar level remains relatively stable, within a certain range, because the insulin is produced efficiently and in just the right quantity to transport glucose to cells for storage. Exercise, stress, infection, food, and sleep all affect these levels, but the blood-sugar level should never rise or fall above or below the normal range.

Insulin isn't the only hormone responsible for the metabolism of sugar and its use by the body. The pancreas also produces *glucagon*, which is used to break down and release the glucose that is stored in the liver. This liver-based glucose, called *glycogen*, serves as fuel for the body. When it is broken down and released from the liver, it raises blood-sugar levels.

So here is what happens when you eat a piece of bread or a candy bar, both of which contain *carbohydrates*. All carbohydrates, whether simple or complex, ultimately break down into their fundamental building block—glucose. The digestive process begins in your mouth, as your saliva starts to break down the carbohydrates. When the food lands in your stomach, it is broken down by the enzymes in your stomach juices. The glucose is absorbed across the intestinal wall into your body and eventually enters your bloodstream. Some of it is used right away. Additional chemicals combine with the glucose, breaking it down yet further into *adenosine triphosphate* (ATP), a chemical used in conjunction with oxygen as an energy source.

What happens to the extra glucose that is not used to meet the body's immediate energy needs? It can't hang around in the bloodstream. It has to go someplace—either to be disposed of or to be stored. This is accomplished by insulin, which transports it into liver and muscle cells. Then later, when energy is needed, the pancreas releases glucagon. This is the chemical responsible for "freeing" the stored glucose (called glycogen) from the liver and muscles. Once it is released back into the blood, the conversion to ATP takes place again and energy is made available.

Type 1 and Type 2 Diabetes

Sometimes, this highly organized and balanced system fails. When the pancreas cannot produce enough insulin because of a built-in defect, this is called *type 1 diabetes*. While it can begin in adulthood, it more often is first diagnosed before the age of nineteen. As a result, it is also referred to as *juvenile-onset diabetes*. Most people with type 1 diabetes must take insulin because the pancreas is incapable of manufacturing this important hormone on its own. Heredity seems to be the most decisive factor here, although lifestyle also plays an important role. The fact that there are individuals with diabetic parents who do *not* go on to develop the disease suggests that, as in most other illnesses, heredity is only one important factor among an array of others that predispose the individual to developing diabetes.

Type 2 diabetes, also called *adult-onset diabetes*, usually strikes older individuals, as the name implies. Typically the illness is diagnosed in people over the age of forty. A person with type 2 diabetes does not start out with a dysfunctional pancreas. In fact, the opposite is true—if you measure the amount of insulin in their bloodstream, you may discover elevated insulin levels, at least in the beginning. The reason for this apparently paradoxical phenomenon is that individuals with type 2 diabetes overload their bodies with so much sugar that the pancreas is forced to keep pumping out the insulin in order to process the extra sugar. As mentioned above, sugar designed to be used fairly quickly by the body as fuel is stored in the liver and muscle cells. That way, when you are engaged in strenuous physical activity, the glycogen is readily available to be mobilized for energy. But these liver and muscle storage cells can become desensitized and can "refuse" to accept any additional supplies of glucose. This happens when the insulin receptors along the cell wall become saturated with insulin and can receive no more. The cells reject the insulin, which continues to float around the bloodstream. This is a prediabetic condition known as *insulin resistance*.

So now we have a great deal of extra sugar in the bloodstream. Its presence sends an urgent message to the pancreas to produce more insulin so as to cart the sugar away. But the insulin is helpless because it has nowhere to "dump" all that extra sugar. Nor can the sugar be used for extra energy. There is only so much energy conversion that can take place in the bloodstream at any given time. Additional energy conversion takes place on a cellular level that requires the presence of certain body chemicals within the cell, as well as other mechanisms of the cell, to complete the chemical reaction. So the massive outpouring of insulin is wasted because the sugar is still at large. Meanwhile, the pancreas continues to receive SOS requests to produce still more insulin because of the large quantities of sugar. And so the vicious cycle continues.

Eventually, the exhausted pancreas becomes incapable of generating more insulin. It starts to fail, and the person develops *dysglycemia,* or glucose intolerance, the next step in the development of diabetes. But because the pancreas has the capability of producing insulin and has simply been overtaxed, this type of diabetes can more easily be controlled by dietary changes, weight loss, and exercise. Fewer people with type 2 diabetes become insulin-dependent compared with those with type 1 diabetes.

What's scary is that this avoidable, lifestyle-induced condition is growing steadily in this country. A 2002 study conducted by Dr. Frank Hu at the Harvard University School of Public Health estimated that the number of people with diabetes could increase by 29 million over the next fifty years as the population fond of junk food and prone to obesity ages. Type 2 diabetes is definitely on the rise and is being diagnosed in younger people today—with terribly detrimental effects on the cardiovascular system.

Although everyone who is overweight or eats large quantities of junk food is at risk, there are certain known factors that increase a person's vulnerability to developing type 2 diabetes. These include the following:

- Obesity—being 20 percent above your ideal body weight, or having a body mass index (BMI) higher than 27 (more about this in chapter 6)
- Family history of diabetes—having a grandparent, parent, or sibling who has or had the condition
- Ethnic background—African-Americans, Alaskan natives, American Indians, Asian Americans, Latinos, and Pacific Islanders are more likely than members of other groups to develop diabetes
- Having developed gestational diabetes (diabetes during pregnancy)
- Having given birth to a baby weighing more than 9 pounds
- Having blood pressure higher than 140/90
- An HDL cholesterol level of less than 35
- A triglyceride level greater than 250

If you fall into any of these categories, you must be especially vigilant.

The Fat Connection

Now let's take a closer look at the transition from insulin resistance to the development of type 2 diabetes. As we saw earlier, insulin production begins to decline. Glucose begins to build up in the body but cannot be used efficiently as a source of fuel. Some gets excreted in the urine. Testing the urine for blood sugar is often the first and easiest method of diagnosing diabetes. However, some of the sugar ends up getting converted into fat and stored in that form in the body.

Sugar stored in muscle and liver cells takes the form of *glycerides*. Sugar stored in fat cells, on the other hand, is stored as *triglycerides*. As the name implies, triglycerides consist of one molecule of glycerol joined to three molecules of fatty acids. These are necessary because they are stored for long-term use. The body needs a certain amount of fat reserves in case of a "rainy day." If there is a famine, these storehouses can be opened and the fat can be used as fuel by being progressively broken down. The first step is the removal of one glyceride molecule, yielding a *diglyceride*. When the next molecule is removed, the substance becomes a *monoglyceride* and eventually a *monoglycerol,* which can be easily converted into fuel.

But too much fat leads to diabetes because the large volume of triglycerides cannot be efficiently absorbed by the body and continues to circulate in the blood. It would seem as though the presence of extra insulin and extra triglycerides in the blood should lead to increased energy, but this is not the case. Remember that the body reaches a certain saturation point—only a limited amount of energy can be produced within the cells. The remaining sugar cannot be converted to energy and remains at large, leading to insulin resistance and, eventually, to burnout on the part of the pancreas. As insulin levels drop, the liver and muscle cells no longer have usable fuel. The individual becomes exhausted and fatigued. The body calls upon stored energy from fat.

One of the typical symptoms of uncontrolled diabetes is extreme thirst. That's because the body always struggles to maintain a state of even balance and sameness, called *homeostasis*. When blood becomes too highly concentrated with a substance such as sugar or salt, the body seeks to dilute the blood so as to restore even balance. It draws liquid from surrounding body tissues, leaving the person thirsty. The extra thirst leads to extra fluid consumption; the extra fluid leads to excess urination, which in turn creates even greater thirst. The person has now developed a full-blown case of type 2 diabetes.

Diabetes and Cardiovascular Disease

People with diabetes have at least double the risk for developing CVD. In fact, heart disease ultimately kills almost 80 percent of people with diabetes in the United States. Adults with diabetes have a death rate from heart disease or stroke that is about two to four times higher than that for adults without diabetes! What's the connection? Vascular disease in particular is highly destructive to people with diabetes, who know that an injury to an extremity (such as a finger or toe) can potentially be deadly because the circulatory system is too weak to deliver the necessary immune substances to heal the injury. Necrosis (tissue death) can set in quickly, resulting in a condition called *gangrene* and often necessitating amputation.

Why is the circulatory system of people with diabetes so sluggish? What makes diabetes so destructive to cardiovascular health? Scientists are still piecing together the puzzle, but they have reached the conclusion that individuals with diabetes have more free radicals at large in their bloodstream than do healthy individuals. These free radicals cause oxidation of the small, dense LDL particles, which then enter the endothelium, leading to endothelial dysfunction. The endothelium is also damaged by a tendency of sympathetic nervous systems of diabetic people to release more of substances called *catecholamines*. These naturally occurring chemicals are instrumental in increasing the constriction of blood vessels, stimulating the heart rate, and increasing blood pressure during times of exercise or crisis. The repeated constriction of blood vessels and raising of blood pressure places a great toll on the delicate endothelial lining. As if this weren't enough, diabetes also causes an increased incidence of plaque instability because the endothelium is continually being asked to tighten up. Moreover, the insulin imbalances in diabetes actually cause an increase in LDL cholesterol and a decrease in HDL cholesterol.

Additionally, when a person has diabetes, blood-sugar levels are often elevated, making the blood thicker and more viscous. The blood doesn't flow as efficiently, so the extremities are unable to receive sufficient supplies of oxygen. This overtaxes and weakens the heart, which must pump harder so that oxygen reaches every part of the body.

Insulin resistance also has been linked to CVD. The insulin stimulates the formation of fat cells in arterial tissue—after all, those triglycerides need someplace to go! They circulate in the blood, but they like to find a "home" for themselves, and often that home is right in the arterial walls. It is interesting that the mechanism of transport for triglycerides is VLDL, which is every bit as destructive. It pads the artery with undesirable layers of fat, making it less elastic and also leading to a narrower lumen with reduced blood flow. Elevated insulin levels also decrease the process of fibrinolysis (breaking down of clotting proteins), thereby thickening the blood and increasing the chances of thrombosis (blood clots) in the heart.

Insulin resistance and diabetes are among the cluster of factors commonly associated with syndrome X, or metabolic syndrome. Typically, these blood-sugar disorders go hand in hand with hypertension, obesity, elevated triglyceride and LDL levels, low HDL cholesterol levels, and excessive midbody fat. All of these conditions can be addressed using the DEAR program outlined in part 2—dietary modification, exercise, additional supplementation, and relaxation.

 Obesity:
Not Just a Cosmetic Problem

"But wait a bit," the Oyster cried,
"Before we have our chat;
For some of us are out of breath,
And all of us are fat!"
—LEWIS CARROLL

Americans are obsessed with weight. Open any magazine, turn on the television, or look at billboards along the side of the road and you will see that "thin is in" and fat is considered unattractive. Gone are the days when plump women were considered beautiful. Our little girls are raised with the impossibly big-busted but otherwise emaciated Barbie as their beauty ideal. There are dozens if not hundreds of fad diets that pop up and disappear regularly, together with a host of medications and supplements designed to "burn fat," speed the metabolism, and produce rapid, quick-fix weight loss. It is sad that so many beautiful people—men as well as women—consider themselves ugly because they do not conform to these absurd standards of attractiveness.

However, obesity is not just a cosmetic problem, but a serious health problem as well. It is ironic that in a country where the beauty ideal is becoming slimmer every day, the population is actually growing heavier.

Recent estimates indicate that nearly 60 percent of the adult population in the United States is now considered obese—up from 50 percent in 1997—and close to one in every three American children is overweight. According to the National Institute of Diabetes and Digestive and Kidney Diseases (NIDDK) of the National Institutes of Health (NIH), the percentage of overweight American children and adolescents (ages six through eleven) has risen alarmingly during recent decades, from 5 percent in the 1960s and 1970s to 11 percent in 1994, to 13 percent in 1999. Among older children and adolescents (ages twelve through nineteen), the percentage was even higher—a staggering 14 percent were obese. All of these children are at high risk for developing cardiovascular disease later in life.

CVD is not the only condition triggered by obesity. Hypertension, type 2 diabetes, and several forms of cancer also are associated with excessive weight. While hypertension is rare in young children, diabetes is becoming more common. Further, research has demonstrated that fat cells are accumulated during childhood and are virtually never eliminated, even if the individual loses weight as an adult. The fat content in the cells may diminish, but the cells always remain, predisposing the person to regaining the weight in the future.

What Is Obesity?

We have an array of colloquial words (some descriptive, others euphemistic) to describe the overweight individual, including obese, fat, king- or queen-sized, plump, and heavy, but actually the only accurate scientific terms are *overweight* and *obese*. Both have specific meanings. NIDDK defines overweight and obesity as excess body weight from muscle, bone, body fluid, or fat. So people who say "I'm not fat, I just have big bones" may be telling the truth! And a person who is bloated due to fluid retention (obviously not a healthy condition, but not obesity either) does not have excessive levels of fat.

Both overweight and obese individuals have weight that is higher than normal for their height. These variables—height and weight—combine to determine your *body mass index,* or BMI. According to the NIH and the Centers for Disease Control and Prevention (CDC), overweight is defined as a BMI of 25 to 29.9 and obesity as a BMI of 30 or greater.

BMI values apply to men and women over age eighteen. However, your BMI may not accurately reflect your body fitness (or fatness)—for example, if you are pregnant or nursing, a competitive athlete or body builder, or a frail elderly person. If you fall into one of these categories, you need to speak to your health-care provider to help you adjust your BMI to more accurately reflect your real body mass index.

BODY MASS INDEX

Your BMI is calculated by dividing your weight in pounds by height in inches squared (multiplied by itself) and then multiplying the result by 703, as follows:

$$\frac{\text{weight (pounds)}}{\text{height (inches)} \times \text{height (inches)}} \times 703 = \text{BMI}$$

Here's an example. Let's say you weigh 210 pounds and are 70 inches (5 feet 10 inches) tall:

$$\frac{210}{70 \times 70} = \frac{210}{4900} = 0.04285 \times 703 = 30.12$$

If you are are not mathematically inclined, however, you can consult table 6.1, which will help you determine your BMI.

Table 6.1 • Estimating Your BMI

BMI	19	20	21	22	23	24	25	26	27	28	29	30	35	40
Height (inches)							Weight (pounds)							
58	91	96	100	105	110	115	119	124	129	134	138	143	167	191
59	94	99	104	109	114	119	124	128	133	138	143	148	173	198
60	97	102	107	112	118	123	128	133	138	143	148	153	179	201
61	100	106	111	116	122	127	132	137	143	148	153	158	185	211
62	104	109	115	120	126	131	136	142	147	158	163	169	197	225
63	107	113	118	124	130	135	141	146	152	158	163	169	197	225
64	110	116	122	128	134	140	145	151	157	163	169	174	204	232
65	114	120	126	132	138	144	150	156	162	168	174	180	210	240
66	118	124	130	136	142	148	155	161	167	173	179	186	216	247
67	121	127	134	140	146	153	159	166	172	178	185	191	223	255
68	125	131	138	144	151	158	164	171	177	184	190	197	230	262
69	128	135	142	149	155	162	169	176	182	189	196	203	236	270
70	132	139	146	153	160	167	174	181	188	195	202	207	243	278
71	136	143	150	157	165	172	179	186	193	200	208	215	250	286
72	140	147	154	162	169	177	184	191	199	206	213	221	258	294
73	144	151	159	166	174	182	189	197	204	212	219	227	265	302
74	148	155	163	171	179	186	194	202	210	218	225	233	272	311
75	152	160	168	176	184	192	200	208	216	224	232	240	279	319
76	156	164	172	180	189	197	205	213	221	230	238	246	287	328

Obviously, this chart is just an approximation. If you want an exact calculation and have Internet access, you can visit http://www.consumer.gov/weightloss.bmi.htm, a government site with a computerized calculator that computes your precise BMI.

APPLES VERSUS PEARS

An additional factor that has a bearing on the degree of risk posed by obesity is the distribution of fat. If fat is accumulated around the waistline—something especially common in middle-aged and older men—it poses a greater health hazard than it would if accumulated elsewhere. An "apple-shaped" person is at great risk. Women tend to be more "pear-shaped"—the weight flares around the abdomen, hips, and buttocks—which is somewhat less problematic. Experts have agreed that a waistline of 40 inches or more in a man and 35 inches in a woman augments weight-related risk.

Why Is It Risky to Be Overweight?

The first issue is a simple matter of physics and gravity. When there is more weight to lug around, the heart must work harder. The extra exertion demands extra exertion by your heart. This may be why it is detrimental to carry most of your weight in the abdominal region. When weight is evenly distributed, it's easier to carry around. However, this is not the primary reason that being overweight is harmful. A large-framed person with big bones or an athlete with bulging muscles does not have increased health risk due to being heavier than average. The concerns are the chemical composition of the fat cells and their impact on the body.

We generally associate fat with what happens when we eat a fattening food—say, a cheeseburger. The fat in the food introduces fat into our bodies. That fat eventually ends up in our cells, and the cholesterol lines our arterial walls. This is true, of course, but an oversimplification. It does not take into account that fat itself emits cytokines, the chemicals associated with inflammation. When we recall the role of inflammation in CVD, we begin to understand more clearly where obesity fits into the picture.

The extra fat cells release extra cytokines. These increase the levels of LDL cholesterol and decrease the levels of HDL cholesterol, which in turn diminishes the elasticity of the blood vessel walls, promoting hypertension. According to a recent analysis conducted by the National Health and Nutrition Examination Survey (NHANES) III, the higher your BMI, the higher your total cholesterol and blood pressure will be. Your HDL cholesterol levels are inversely related to your BMI, meaning that the lower your BMI, the higher your HDL cholesterol will be, and vice versa.

The findings are sobering. Men with the highest BMI had more than twice the average risk of developing high blood pressure and high cholesterol. Women with the highest BMI had four times the risk! Autopsies of young men (ages fifteen to thirty-four) who died of non-CVD-related causes revealed fatty streaks, plaque, and raised atherosclerotic lesions in their right coronary arteries, and smaller lesions elsewhere. Those with high BMIs consistently showed higher levels of these early signs of atherosclerosis and inflammation than those who were less obese.

These pre-atherosclerotic and pre-inflammatory signs begin even earlier than mid-adolescence. An international study of 3,512 children between eight and sixteen years old showed elevated blood concentrations of C-reactive protein and elevated white blood cell counts in the obese children, findings that point to the presence of inflammation.

Scientists have begun to regard obesity as especially dangerous when it appears as a component of syndrome X, or the metabolic syndrome. In this condition, obesity goes hand in hand with elevated cholesterol, elevated triglycerides, and hypertension. In fact, the NCEP-ATP III pointed to the importance of addressing the metabolic syndrome by offering patients intensified treatment to reduce obesity. The focus on weight loss is one component of the revised guidelines issued by the NCEP-ATP III. As I continue to treat patients over the years, I become more and more convinced that obesity leads to more chronic health problems than any other single factor except, perhaps, cigarette smoking.

The Ups and Downs of Obesity

Here's another reason why obesity stresses the heart. Many (if not most) overweight individuals go on a series of diets, only to regain the weight later. This so-called yo-yo dieting effect takes a great toll on the entire system, including the heart. Each time you lose weight, you decrease the amount of fat not only in your fat cells but also in your muscle cells. (Remember that some fat is needed to repair and maintain muscle cells, and that some cholesterol is actually manufactured in these cells.) So there is a reduction in lean muscle mass that accompanies a reduction in fat tissue. The more rapid your weight loss, the greater your muscle loss. True, you may be losing pounds and may jump off the scale joyously. But actually, you are losing more muscle than fatty tissue. This isn't healthy. You need muscles for all kinds of reasons—and ironically, the more muscle mass you have, the higher your metabolic body rate, meaning that you burn fat more quickly. When you lose muscle, your metabolic rate slows down.

What happens when your metabolic rate slows? For one thing, your weight loss also slows down, leading to the well-known "plateau" that is the undoing of so many zealous dieters. They reach a point at which they are still starving themselves but are no longer losing weight. Their metabolism is working against them. Even more disturbing, when they start to overeat again (as so many do), they regain the weight as *fat,* not as muscle! In fact, they never regain the muscle mass that has been lost during their crash diet. They're stuck with extra fat tissue and a slower metabolism as well, making their next foray into the weight-loss jungle even more difficult. They end up in a cycle in which they lose muscle mass and substitute fat, then lose more muscle mass and gain more fat, and so on, which places increasingly greater stress upon the cardiovascular system. The cycle also depletes important nutrients from the body.

So no matter how obese my patients might be, I always advise them to lose no more than one to two pounds a week. This is both physically and psychologically sound. It makes it possible for people to establish new eating patterns that can be sustained, rather than enduring heroic bouts of asceticism and starvation that are bound to wear out quickly. They are less likely to start overeating again and regaining the weight. More important, they will lose fat, not muscle. And in general, I always advise patients to make changes gradually because the body craves homeostasis, and stress is created on the body to be abruptly wrenched from one state to another. A slower process is gentler for the whole system.

If you follow the dietary suggestions outlined in part 2 of this book, you will lose weight, but in a *healthy* way, and hopefully you will also be able to keep the weight off. But diet is not enough. It is known that a sedentary lifestyle contributes to obesity because the body cannot burn off the calories taken in through the excessive food. I also provide you with an exercise program that can address your weight in a gradual and healthy way.

7 Your Heart Goes Up in Smoke

My days have crackled and gone up in smoke.
—Francis Thompson

Barney was forty-two years old when he was admitted to the hospital with chest pain that turned out to be a heart attack. There was no family history of cardiovascular disease, and Barney's checkups had been normal. Although he led a sedentary life and was slightly overweight, he appeared to be in good health. In fact, he had virtually no cardiovascular risk factors beyond gender and sedentary lifestyle. The mystery was quickly solved when it emerged that Barney was a heavy smoker—two to three packs each day. He was surprised when he found out that smoking was probably the main cause of his heart attack. "I could understand lung cancer," he told me, "but what do cigarettes have to do with the heart?"

Barney is not alone. A disturbingly small number of people are aware of the connection between cigarette smoking and cardiovascular disease. Yet in the United States, 400,000 deaths each year can be attributed to smoking—that's about 1,200 deaths per day—and it is estimated that at least one-third of these deaths are related to CVD. That is an absolutely staggering number. Responding to this alarming state of affairs, the surgeon general has called cigarette smoking the most important of the known modifiable risk factors for coronary artery disease in the United States.

It amazes me that many people are not more aware of this connection. Many also have misconceptions about smoking. They think that low-tar cigarettes are less detrimental than other cigarettes, or that using a filter can reduce the risk. This simply isn't true. All cigarette smoke is an assault on the cardiovascular system. Let's understand why.

Smoke Signals

To begin with, tobacco smoke contains approximately four thousand substances. We don't even know all the chemicals that are being introduced to the body with every cigarette a person smokes. We do know that nicotine, tar, and hydrocarbons have the most deleterious effects—but this does not mean that the other substances in the smoke are innocuous. Any foreign material can cause damage to the body.

Cigarette smoke causes direct damage to the endothelial lining of your arteries by introducing free radicals to the system. Remember that these chemicals are known to cause oxidative damage. Usually we think of oxygen as a good thing, and with good reason. Every time we eat or breathe, our cells undergo oxidation. This is a normal metabolic process. One of the by-products of this process, however, is the formation of free radicals—waste products given off by our cells in the course of healthy oxidation. Think of what happens to an apple when it is cut open and its interior exposed to oxygen. The white surface becomes brown. Think of what happens when iron rusts. The brown on the apple and the rust on the iron are both by-products of oxidation.

Free radicals can wreak havoc in the arterial wall by disrupting the delicate surface structure, setting the stage for the entrance of fat cells and the development of plaque. They also elevate levels of fibrinogen, raising the risk of heart attack and stroke. In the normal course of events, the free radicals are disposed of by other substances, called *antioxidants*. The normal process of oxidation remains in balance with the disposal of wastes, and you remain healthy. However, if you introduce extraordinarily large quantities of free radicals into the body, its natural mechanisms cannot cope with them all, and oxidative damage results.

Smoking and Blood Pressure

There are additional reasons why smoking contributes to CVD. When you inhale cigarette smoke, the nicotine increases your blood pressure and heart rate. Within one minute of inhaling the first puff, the heart rate begins to rise. It can increase by as much as 30 percent during the first ten minutes of smoking. The blood pressure rises, the blood vessels constrict, and the heart pumps harder and harder. This is part of the pleasant "rush" people experience when they inhale cigarette smoke. They feel energized. But this increase in blood pressure happens at a terrible price. Smoking potentiates (increases) the effects of hypertension. Additionally, if you take antihypertensive medication, smoking will reduce its effectiveness.

Carbon Monoxide Poisoning

Here's a little-known fact about cigarette smoke: It contains carbon monoxide—yes, the same lethal gas that's found in car exhaust. When it is released into your bloodstream, carbon monoxide reduces the amount of oxygen that your blood can carry to your organs by constricting the arteries, especially in the extremities (arms and legs). Remember that cigarette smoke has a *vasoconstrictive* effect—that is, it tightens the lumen of the blood vessel, making less room available for blood flow.

But carbon monoxide has an even more destructive effect. It attaches itself to hemoglobin more easily than oxygen does. This is why it is possible to commit suicide with car exhaust—hemoglobin cells "choose" available carbon monoxide over available oxygen, and the body becomes starved of oxygen in a short period of time because the hemoglobin cannot accept oxygen. The result is a diminution of the blood's ability to deliver oxygen to the organs in the body. This is most detrimental during exercise, when the heart is demanding more oxygen. Now we have a heart that's working harder at the very time that the oxygen supply is decreasing. This causes a condition known as *ischemia*—a lack of oxygen and blood flow to the tissues, including the heart muscle. If the arteries have already been narrowed by deposits of plaque, the condition is even more dangerous.

This is why smokers with angina (chest pains due to atherosclerosis) experience chest pains so quickly when they exercise. The constant influx of cigarette smoke has reduced the amount of oxygen supplied to the heart and has also forced the heart to beat faster.

But in case you think that this condition only affects people with atherosclerosis, let me add that even normal coronary arteries can go into spasm and cause ischemia while you are smoking. You may not experience chest pain, but the constriction of the arteries certainly takes place. It is exacerbated by exercise, because smoking blocks the increased blood flow that normally occurs during exercise, so the cells in the body as well as the heart do not get the extra oxygen they need to compensate for the extra exertion.

The heart and coronary arteries are the most significantly affected by smoking, but the damaging effects of cigarette smoke do not stop there. Smoking also contributes to peripheral vascular disease. In fact, smokers have a sixteenfold increased risk for developing this condition, in which the blood vessels leading to the arms and legs become narrow due to atherosclerotic plaque buildup. This condition can lead to intermittent claudication (pain in the legs due to insufficient oxygen supply to the muscles). Extremely severe cases of ongoing claudication can eventually lead to destruction of the skin or muscle tissue that is continually deprived of oxygen.

Finally, smoking contributes to other diseases, such as chronic bronchitis and emphysema. These lung conditions, which diminish the overall oxygen supply in the body, force the heart to work still harder to transport the available oxygen to all the needed locations. And smoking can interact poorly with medications. It reduces the effectiveness of angina medication, for example. And it is well known that the combination of cigarettes and birth control pills raises the risk of stroke.

But I'm Not a Heavy Smoker!

One does not have to be a heavy smoker to suffer the ill effects of smoking. Even a few cigarettes can be quite damaging. Earlier, we alluded to the well-known Framingham Study, which followed over 5,000 individuals (2,282 men and 2,845 women) culled from the general population over a fourteen-year period. One of the findings demonstrated an increase in mortality due to CVD of 18 percent in men and 31 percent in women for every ten cigarettes smoked each day. These findings have been corroborated by numerous other studies, both within the United States and worldwide.

I hope that I have convinced you that the pleasant feelings you might get from smoking are not worth the enormous risks and health hazards you are taking every time you put a cigarette into your mouth. If you need to relax or want to feel a mild rush of energy, there are much safer ways to achieve these goals. We will discuss those in chapter 14.

 Other Risk Factors for Cardiovascular Disease

For the blood is the spirit.
—Leviticus

I have grouped several apparently unrelated risk factors into a single chapter. Some, like age and family history, are beyond your control. This chapter is designed to inform you of the risks associated with these, but cannot offer solutions. The awareness of other risk factors—such as infections—is only now emerging in the scientific community. There is still relatively little research corroborating these findings—not enough to warrant an entire chapter. But this book would not be complete without mention of these new areas of exploration. So they are included in this chapter as well.

Gender

The difference between the risk of men and women has long been part of popular consciousness. In fact, many people believe that the typical heart attack victim is male and that women are, for the most part, immune to cardiovascular disease. Men do have a higher incidence of CVD than women do, and the disease usually develops about ten years earlier in men than in women. Being male increases the risk of developing CVD because men do not produce nearly as much estrogen as women do. Estrogen, a female sex hormone, has a protective effect on the arterial walls. It helps the arteries to dilate so that blood flow is increased by enhancing the function of *endothelial derived relaxing factor* (EDRF), which relaxes the arterial walls. It also protects the endothelium from oxidative damage. Obviously, estrogen is produced only in tiny quantities by the male hormonal system. However, this does not mean that men are completely defenseless. A recent Dutch study of 6,732 individuals over age fifty-five found that those with higher testosterone levels had a lower incidence of stroke. The study included female participants as well and found that those women with higher testosterone levels sustained fewer strokes than those with lower levels. Needless to say, this would give men an edge over women as far as the risk of stroke is concerned. Here's a fascinating additional finding of the study: Higher testosterone levels provided no protection whatsoever for smokers, male or female. Of course, as you age, testosterone levels drop. This may be one aspect of the network of factors that raise the risk of CVD as people age.

Although women reach the age of maximum risk about ten years later than men do, more women than men die of CVD on an annual basis. In fact, cardiovascular disease is the leading cause of death in women and more destructive than the next fourteen causes of death combined! Even more disturbing, most women discount their risk. A recent survey conducted by the American Heart Association found that only 8 percent of women interviewed cited heart disease as their leading health threat, compared with more than 50 percent who worried about cancer. The reality is quite different from their perception—only one in twenty-eight women will die of breast cancer, while one in two women will die of CVD.

Why the ignorance? Because at younger ages, women *do* have a lower incidence of heart disease due to the presence of estrogen in their bodies. As mentioned above, estrogen has a protective effect on the endothelial lining of the artery. But as women age, they lose this protective hormone. During menopause, estrogen levels drop dramatically, resulting in hot flashes, mood swings, and other unpleasant experiences associated with menopause, and ultimately resulting in the complete cessation of menstrual periods.

Once a woman's body is no longer producing sufficient quantities of estrogen, she loses the protection it offered and becomes more vulnerable to CVD. Because of this, it was once standard practice for doctors to recommend hormone replacement therapy (HRT) with estrogen for postmenopausal women. It was widely believed that this would protect women from CVD, and some studies appeared to support that contention. But the safety and efficacy of HRT have been severely challenged. HRT has been associated with several types of cancer. In fact, the U.S. government has added synthetic estrogen replacement therapy to its official list of cancer-causing agents.

Despite the association of HRT with cancer, its promoters continued to tout its virtues by claiming that it had beneficial effects on cardiovascular health. It has now emerged, however, that synthetic estrogen replacement therapy actually promotes CVD by increasing the risk of blood clots! The first study to suggest this, called the Heart and Estrogen/Progestin Replacement Study (HERS) was reported in the *Journal of the American Medical Association* in 1998. More recently, a major study of 28,000 women, called the Women's Health Initiative, was halted in midstudy due to the detrimental cardiovacular effects of estrogen replacement.

What is the reason for the disturbing increase in heart attack, stroke, and blood clots among postmenopausal women on HRT? Researchers are not sure, but it has been hypothesized that HRT is associated with increased levels of C-reactive protein. It therefore appears that HRT does its damage by increasing inflammation. And while scientists are not sure why naturally occurring estrogen protects the arteries, while synthetic estrogen damages the arteries, one thing is clear—postmenopausal women must find different ways to protect themselves against CVD.

If I've scared you, then I have done my job. I want to shake you out of the complacency I so often see in my female patients and make you realize that once women are past menopause, cardiovascular disease is an equal opportunity afflicter!

Age

The percentage of individuals with CVD increases with age, with most heart attacks affecting people over the age of sixty-five. While scientists have not fully determined why the aging process itself occurs, it appears that the body has a built-in biological clock that begins to run down. The normal wear and tear of daily living affects your body like the wear and tear on anything that gets regular use—your car, your washing machine, your computer. Stressors, such as illnesses or environmental toxins, speed the process by increasing the damage done to your body's organs and systems. By making these organs and systems work harder, they create even more wear and tear. The heart and blood vessels change as people age, even if there is no disease process taking place. The muscle of the heart, like other muscles, becomes less elastic. Its pumping action therefore becomes less efficient, and it must work harder to do the same job. Additionally, the cells of the heart that control its rhythmic beating pattern (called *pacemaker cells*) atrophy and die, leaving the heart at risk of rhythmic irregularities.

The changes caused by aging also affect the walls of your blood vessels, making them less elastic. The decrease in levels of estrogen and testosterone is also responsible for the decrease in the elasticity of the arterial walls. This means they cannot expand and contract efficiently, which places more stress upon the heart.

Family History

Genetics play an important role in the development of any disease process, including that of CVD. We all know that certain tendencies run in families. Sometimes we hear of three generations of men who died of a heart attack in their fifties, or of a daughter who suffered from a stroke when she was just a few years older than her mother had been when she had had one. While we cannot alter our genes, we certainly can become aware of them. I urge my patients to investigate their family histories and familiarize themselves with diseases that run in the family. If your grandmother had angina, you know that you must be even more careful about leading a heart-healthy lifestyle. If an uncle suddenly dropped dead of a heart attack at age forty-five, despite having been told he was fit as a fiddle at his last checkup, you know that he might have been a victim of the silent, insidious process of inflammation, leading to the destabilization of plaque, the rupture of the fibrous cap, and rapid death. The more you know about your family history, the more you know about your own risk factors, and the more motivated you will be to take care of your health.

Medication

Certain medications increase the risk of developing CVD. These include:

- Carbamezapine (Tegretol)
- Colestipol (Cholestid)
- Methotrexate (Rheumatrex)
- Phenytoin (Dilantin)
- Thiazide diuretics
- Oral contraceptives (especially when used in combination with smoking)

If you are taking any of these these drugs, you need to be particularly vigilant about your diet. In fact, I would recommend that you place yourself in the low- to moderate-risk category even if you have no other risk factors (see chapter 9).

Sedentary Lifestyle

Most Americans (probably around 60 percent of the population) are physically inactive, which is highly detrimental to cardiac health. It is well known that exercise decreases the risk of developing CVD and increases good health on many different levels. And studies have associated a sedentary lifestyle with a much higher risk of CVD.

Stress

Stress has been established as one of the most major risk factors for the development of CVD. This has become part of folk wisdom and idiom: "Don't upset your mother, you'll give her a heart attack!" When we're upset, we say that our heart "stood still" or "skipped a beat." This isn't just a poetic metaphor. There are real physiological changes in the heart when we receive bad news, undergo a trauma, or live with stressful situations on an ongoing basis.

Infections

Much interesting new research points to the possible role that certain infections may play in the development of CVD. These infections include the Epstein-Barr virus (EBV), which causes mononucleosis; *Chlamydia pneumoniae* and *Mycoplasma pneumoniae,* two organisms that can cause pneumonia; herpes simplex, the virus that causes mouth ulcers, cold sores, and genital herpes; and *Helicobacter pylori,* a type of bacteria that causes most stomach ulcers.

The exact mechanism by which infections may increase heart disease is unclear. One theory, advanced by Dr. Paul Ridker, director of the Center for Cardiovascular Disease Prevention at Brigham and Women's

Hospital in Boston, suggests that infections do their damage by increasing inflammation in the body. When there is an infection, the body's immune system kicks in to get rid of the infection, but this also aggravates the inflammatory process already taking place in the arteries.

Periodontal Disease

Another new source of interest among scientists for its possible role in the development of CVD is *periodontal disease* (inflammation or infections of the gums around the teeth, such as gingivitis). The theory is that when oral bacteria enter the bloodstream, they trigger the liver to make proteins, such as C-reactive protein, that add to the inflammatory process in the arteries.

# Assessing Your Risk

Know thyself...
— Ancient Greek wisdom

Now that you understand the various risk factors for the development of cardiovascular disease, it's time to look at your own risk. You have probably begun to draw some conclusions already and are wondering what you can do to cut down on your risk factors. We have seen that a risk factor does not guarantee that a problem will develop but rather places you at greater risk for the development of that problem. But how rigorous do you have to be? How can you know if you have a dangerous condition brewing in your bloodstream? How can you determine your level of risk? These are important questions because, as we mentioned in previous chapters, unstable plaque can be a silent killer that ruptures at any time without warning. When this happens, the consequences can be swift and deadly. Even apparently healthy, physically fit young people can be affected. Think of Sergei Grinkov, for example, the Olympic figure skater who suddenly collapsed and died of a heart attack at the age of twenty-eight. Or Darryl Kile, a starting pitcher for the St. Louis Cardinals, who suddenly died of a heart attack at the age of thirty-three. Both athletes had no known health problems.

Having information about the state of your arterial walls will let you know how rigorous you must be in reducing those risk factors over which you have control. I am not suggesting that if your risk is low, you should make saturated fats a dietary staple or neglect to exercise. But how many liberties you can take with your fat consumption and how much exercise you incorporate into your daily routine will be determined, to a large extent, by how serious your risk is. And if you are at high risk, you will need to tackle the problem aggressively, not only by eliminating as many risk factors as possible but also by implementing the DEAR program even more rigorously.

I assess an individual's level of risk by looking not only at one specific risk factor (such as the blood cholesterol level) but rather by taking stock of the global level of risk, based on a combination of *all* risk factors. This is a more helpful and accurate measure of risk than the focus on a single factor. I base my assessment of global risk on a scale that I have created and that I have found extremely useful in my clinical experience. Translating all the myriad risk factors into a set of numbers has helped my patients understand their level of risk and make decisions about diet, supplements, and exercise.

Accordingly, I use system that assigns each risk factor a certain number of points. The higher the point level, the higher your risk. The number of points assigned is based on how serious the risk factor is. For example, smoking is an extremely serious risk factor and is far more alarming than male gender. Your risk level is also based on how much you are out of the range of normal. If you are overweight by five pounds, for example, your risk is lower than if you are overweight by one hundred pounds.

Before we determine your risk, let's briefly review the major risk factors. They fall into two categories: those that are associated with lifestyle or personal or family history, and those that emerge from blood tests.

Lifestyle and personal and family history and other factors include the following:

- Smoking
- Obesity
- Diabetes/insulin resistance
- Hypertension
- Family history of cardiovascular disease
- Personal history of cardiovascular disease
- Male gender/postmenopausal status
- Advanced age
- Sedentary lifestyle
- High-stress lifestyle/type A personality
- Infections

Factors that emerge from blood tests include the following:

- High total cholesterol level
- High LDL cholesterol level
- Low HDL cholesterol level
- High homocysteine level
- High hs-CRP level
- High Lp(a) level
- High triglyceride level
- High fibrinogen level
- High ferritin level

Although we know that a high-stress lifestyle is associated with an increased incidence of CVD, I do not include stress levels in my assessment of risk because they cannot be easily measured. The things that cause stress are as individual as the people who experience them, and perceptions of stress are quite personal and highly subjective. So I ask you to take stock of your own stress levels based on everything in your life that causes *you* stress, whether someone else would call it stressful or not.

Further, whatever level of risk that emerges from your risk profile, you should recognize that stress will potentiate every other risk factor and make the need for aggressive approaches even more urgent.

Like stress, age is a risk factor that I won't quantify. Risk rises with increasing age. Use your good judgment and recognize that the older you are, the greater your risk.

I also do not include infections, fibrinogen levels, or ferritin levels in the assessment of your risk. Although they are recognized risk factors, scientists are still evolving in their understanding of how to assess and quantify their significance. Moreover, these tests are not commonly prescribed (yet). I want to provide you with easily accessible measurements and established guidelines that are used by most physicians. But again, be sensible. If you have received an elevated score on your ferritin or fibrinogen levels, recognize that your risk level is higher than the total you tally upon reading this chapter.

The Risk-Factor Questionnaire

I have found it useful to divide my patients into four groups. In the test that follows, assign a numerical value to each risk factor. If the condition does not apply to you, enter 0. At the end of the questionnaire section, tally up the total and find out where you stand.

- **Smoking.** This is one of the most dangerous activities in which you can engage and therefore one of the most serious risk factors. There is simply no safe level of smoking, so I don't stratify risk based on how many cigarettes you smoke each day. If you smoke, you're at maximum risk:

    Smoking: 6 points   YOUR SCORE: _____

- **Obesity.** Remember that obesity is defined as an elevated BMI. Obviously someone with a slightly elevated BMI is at less risk than someone with a grossly elevated BMI. Here are some guidelines (see the BMI chart on p. 64):

BMI of 25 to 26: 2 points
BMI of 27 to 30: 4 points
BMI over 31: 6 points   YOUR SCORE: _____

- **Diabetes/insulin resistance.** The risk for people with diabetes varies, depending on the degree to which the diabetic condition is under control.

    Insulin resistance: 2 points
    Diabetes, controlled (fasting glucose of 110 to 125): 4 points
    Diabetes, uncontrolled (fasting glucose above 126): 6 points
                                                    YOUR SCORE: _____

- **Hypertension.** This is one of the most significant risk factors for CVD. Your risk rises as your blood pressure rises.

    Systolic pressure of 140 or above and/or
    diastolic pressure of 90 or above: 6 points   YOUR SCORE: _____

- **Family history.** If any immediate family member (parent, grandparent, or sibling) has suffered from a heart attack, stroke, hypertension, high cholesterol, or other signs of CVD, you are also at risk.

    Family history of CVD: 2 points   YOUR SCORE: _____

- **Personal history.** Any history of heart attack or stroke places you at greater risk than a healthy person with no prior history, even if you have taken measures to reduce the risk.

    Personal history of CVD: 3 points   YOUR SCORE: _____

- **Male gender/postmenopausal status.** Remember that men are at greater risk of developing CVD than women because the female sex hormone estrogen confers protective benefit on the artery walls. This is why men as well as postmenopausal women are both at greater risk than premenopausal women.

  Male gender/postmenopausal status: 2 points   YOUR SCORE: _____

- **Sedentary lifestyle.** The absence of exercise is a major risk factor, while engaging in exercise offers significant protective benefits. For this reason, I assign a point value to sedentary lifestyle, based on how little you engage in physical activity. If you exercise, then congratulate yourself. You can deduct some points!

  Completely sedentary: 3 points
  Inconsistent exercise: 2 points
  Consistent exercise (up to 1 hour a week): *subtract* 1 point
  Consistent exercise (1 to 2 hours a week): *subtract* 2 points
  Consistent exercise (more than 2 hours a week):
    subtract 3 points   YOUR SCORE: _____

- **High LDL cholesterol.** As you know, elevated cholesterol is no longer regarded as a single, undifferentiated concept but is divided into several categories, each of which has its own set of risk factors.

  LDL cholesterol below 100 mg/dL: 0 points
  LDL cholesterol between 101 and 129 mg/dL: 2 points
  LDL cholesterol between 130 and 159 mg/dL: 4 points
  LDL cholesterol 160 mg/dL or above: 6 points
                                  YOUR SCORE: _____

- **Low HDL cholesterol.** Remember that HDL ("good") cholesterol confers protective benefits on the cardiovascular system. For this reason, you are rewarded for having high HDL levels by *subtracting* points:

    HDL cholesterol between 60 and 80 mg/dL: *subtract* 1 point
    HDL cholesterol above 81 mg/dL: *subtract* 2 points

    YOUR SCORE: _____

- **Homocysteine.** Homocysteine is emerging as a more serious risk factor than originally thought, and as significant as cholesterol.

    Homocysteine under 10 µmol/L: 0 points
    Homocysteine between 10 and 15 µmol/L: 2 points
    Homocysteine between 16 and 20 µmol/L: 4 points
    Homocysteine 21 µmol/L or above: 6 points

    YOUR SCORE: _____

- **Cardiac-CRP**

    Cardiac-CRP 1 mg/L or below: 0 points
    Cardiac-CRP between 1.01 and 1.5 mg/L: 2 points
    Cardiac-CRP between 1.6 and 2.0 mg/L: 4 points
    Cardiac-CRP 2.01 mg/L or above: 6 points

    YOUR SCORE: _____

- **Lipoprotein (a)**

    Lp(a) 30 mg/dL or below: 0 points
    Lp(a) between 31 and 40 mg/dL: 2 points
    Lp(a) between 41 and 50 mg/dL: 4 points
    Lp(a) 51 mg/dL or above: 6 points

    YOUR SCORE: _____

- **Triglycerides**

    Triglycerides 150 mg/dL or less: 0 points
    Triglycerides between 151 and 200 mg/dL: 2 points
    Triglycerides between 201 and 250 mg/dL: 4 points
    Triglycerides 251 mg/dL or above: 6 points   YOUR SCORE: _____

Now tally up all of your points: **YOUR TOTAL SCORE:** _____

Based on your total score, you can determine which of the following risk-level categories you fit into, and what it means:

- 5 points or less: Level 1 (prevention). This is appropriate for those whose risk is negligible or extremely low. You want to be sure that you never get into any higher-risk category.
- 6 to 10 points: Level 2 (mild risk). You can't be complacent. Your risk may be relatively low, but you still have some concerns. If you address them now, you can head off more serious problems in the future.
- 11 to 15 points: Level 3 (moderate risk). You have to sit up and take notice. You have some significant risk factors and must approach them aggressively.
- 16 points or higher: Level 4 (high risk). It is urgent that you address your health and alter your lifestyle immediately! You are at serious risk and must take the most aggressive measures possible to prevent further damage and reverse already existing damage if possible.

Remember also to take note of additional risk-raising factors that are not quantified, such as stress levels and age. Please also note that you are at higher risk if you have a history of infections or elevated ferritin and/or fibrinogen levels.

Now that you have assessed your risk, we can turn to the DEAR program to see how you can treat your condition and lower your risk for CVD.

PART TWO

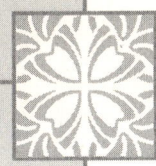

What Can I Do?

The DEAR Program

10 Eating with CARE
Basic Elements of the Diet

> *The doctor of the future will give no medicine but will interest his patients in the care of the human frame, in diet, and in the cause and prevention of disease ... The physician of tomorrow will be the nutritionist of today.*
> —Thomas Edison

This chapter will look at which foods are generally beneficial to eat, and in what proportions. To find out *why* these foods are good for you, refer to "Important Nutrients in the Diet" below. It shows the healthy ingredients in the healthy foods I recommend, with specific focus on those nutrients that are beneficial to cardiovascular health. It is my hope that acquainting yourself with the nutritional content of your food will bolster your commitment to the CARE (coronary artery rehabilitation eating) diet.

Important Nutrients in the Diet

The nutrients in the table below fall into several categories: phytonutrients (healthy substances that come from plant sources), vitamins, minerals, and amino acids. Please note that for each nutritional category, there is extensive scientific documentation of its benefits. Those foods marked with an asterisk represent particularly good sources of the nutrients in question.

Nutrient	Type	Function	Food Sources
Allium	Phytonutrient	Lowers blood pressure Fights infection and inflammation Helps to balance glucose metabolism Helps to reduce cholesterol Helps to thin blood When eaten with meals, mitigates some ill effects of high-cholesterol foods Potentiates the effects of DHA and EPA	Garlic, leeks, onions
Biotin	Vitamin (part of B family)	Metabolizes carbohydrates, proteins, and fats Important for the synthesis of essential fatty acids	Agar, dark green vegetables, egg yolks, fish (especially sardines), kidney, liver, milk, soybeans, whole grains
Calcium	Mineral	Strengthens bones and teeth Regulates muscle contractions Regulates nerve impulses and hormones	Almonds, apricots (dried), artichokes, beans (green, lima, mung, pinto, red, and white), beet greens, black currants, Brazil nuts, broccoli,

Nutrient	Type	Function	Food Sources
Calcium *(continued)*	Mineral	Assists in blood clotting May help to lower blood pressure	Brussels sprouts, cabbage, carrots, cashews, celery, chestnuts, chickpeas (garbanzos), chicory, Chinese cabbage (bok choy), chives, collard greens*, dairy products, dandelion greens, dates*, elderberries, endive, figs*, filberts (hazelnuts), kale*, kelp, kohlrabi, kumquats, leeks, lentils, lettuce (especially dark green varieties), macadamia nuts, mustard greens,* okra, olives, oranges, parsley, parsnips, peaches (dried), peas, pecans, prunes,* pumpkin, raisins, rhubarb, rice, rutabaga, rye grain, salmon, sardines (with the bones),* scallions, sea vegetables (agar,* arame, dulse,* hijiki,* kombu,* nori,* and wakame*), sesame seeds,* shallots, shrimp, soybeans,*

Nutrient	Type	Function	Food Sources
Calcium *(continued)*	Mineral		soymilk,* spinach, squash, sunflower seeds, Swiss chard, tangerines, tofu,* turnip greens, turnips, walnuts, wheat
Capsaicin	Phytonutrient	Acts as an antioxidant	Hot peppers
Choline and inositol	Vitamins (part of B family)	Help to metabolize, utilize, and absorb cholesterol/fat	Egg yolks, fruits, milk, organ meats, soybeans, vegetables, whole grains
Chromium	Mineral	Helps to metabolize glucose Helps to metabolize fatty acids and cholesterol Helps with insulin regulation by keeping insulin in balance so that excess quantities do not circulate through the bloodstream	Beans, black pepper, brewer's yeast, cheese, meat, mushrooms, peanuts, whole grains
Copper	Mineral	Assists in bone and blood formation Helps to maintain connective tissue Lowers cholesterol levels Helps to regulate arrhythmias	Avocado, cauliflower, dried beans, dried peas, leafy green vegetables, legumes, nuts, shellfish (especially oysters), whole grains
Coumarins	Phytonutrients	Prevent blood clotting	Beans, citrus fruits, grains, nuts, parsley, tomatoes

Nutrient	Type	Function	Food Sources
Flavonoids	Phytonutrients	Impart pigment to brightly colored fruits and vegetables Act as antioxidants Fight LDL buildup and inflammation Strengthen blood vessel walls Improve endothelial function Lower blood pressure Help blood vessel walls to relax	Berries, carrots, citrus fruits, grape skins, kale, onions, peppers, red wine, tea (green and ordinary black), tomatoes
Genistein	Phytoestrogen	Protects endothelium from damage after menopause when estrogen levels drop Boosts estrogen levels	Chickpeas (garbanzo beans), lentils, soybeans
Glutathione	Amino acid consisting of three amino acids: cystine, glutamic acid, and glycine	Acts as an antioxidant Neutralizes free radicals Protects against environmental illness, cancer, autoimmune disorders, eye disease, and CVD	Acorn squash, asparagus, avocado, Brussels sprouts, cabbage, eggs, fresh fruit, grapefruit, kale, lean meats, potatoes, strawberries, watermelon, wheat germ, whole grains
Indoles	Phytonutrients	Protect against some female cancers by modulating estrogen metabolism Contain potent antioxidants	Broccoli, Brussels sprouts, cabbage, kale

Nutrient	Type	Function	Food Sources
Indoles *(continued)*	Phytonutrients	Are high in fiber Might help to protect against CVD	
Iron	Mineral	Crucial for the formation of red blood cells and maintaining hemoglobin levels	Eggs, fish, green leafy vegetables, legumes, liver, meat, molasses, poultry, sea vegetables, whole grains
Isoflavones	Phytonutrients	Protect against CVD Protect against osteoporosis and some cancers Modulate estrogens Help to oxidize LDL cholesterol Help to lower homocysteine levels Lower high blood pressure	Chickpeas (garbanzo beans), legumes, soy products (miso, tempeh, and tofu)
Lignans	Phytoestrogens	Act as strong antioxidants Modulate estrogen levels Have mild cholesterol-lowering properties Benefit people with diabetes	Barley, flaxseeds, sea vegetables (dried), sesame seeds, soybeans, wheat
Lycopene	Phytonutrient	Acts as an antioxidant Helps to reduce LDL cholesterol Protects against heart attacks	Papaya, pink grapefruit, pink guava, red grapefruit, strawberries, tomatoes, watermelon

Nutrient	Type	Function	Food Sources
Magnesium	Mineral	Helps in absorption of calcium Facilitates at least 300 different enzymes in the body Facilitates the production of ATP, which is necessary for energy production Helps to regulate heartbeat rhythm Relaxes smooth muscle Helps with vasodilation Acts as a natural calcium-channel blocker Is especially important for people with diabetes, who tend to be deficient in it	Bananas, dried beans and peas, green vegetables, nuts, seafood, sea vegetables, whole grains
Manganese	Mineral	Helps to maintain normal bone density Plays a role in sex hormone production Helps to build healthy cartilage and nerves Is important for glucose metabolism (low levels can cause abnormal glucose metabolism, which can adversely affect the arterial endothelium and contribute to the inflammatory process)	Avocado, celery, dried beans, nuts, peas, sea vegetables, whole grains
Para-amino-benzoic acid (PABA)	Vitamin (part of B family)	Aids in metabolism of protein and folic acid	Dark green vegetables, eggs, kidney, liver, molasses, whole grains, yogurt

Nutrient	Type	Function	Food Sources
Phosphorus	Mineral	Helps to metabolize calcium, vitamins, proteins, carbohydrates, and fats Is vital for healthy bones and teeth Assists in tissue growth and repair	Dairy products, eggs, fish, legumes, meat, nuts, poultry, sea vegetables (arame, dulse, hijiki, kombu, nori, wakame), seeds, whole grains
Polyphenols	Phytonutrients	Inhibit the production of endothelin-1, which contributes to atherosclerosis A member of a class of proteins known as peptides, endothelin-1 is a powerful vasoconstrictor Inhibit LDL oxidation	Broccoli, cranberries, ginger, grape juice, nuts (especially walnuts), oranges, red wine
Potassium	Mineral	Regulates water and sodium balance Regulates nervous and hormonal systems Helps muscles to contract Helps to regulate blood pressure Protects against cardiac arrhythmias Is essential for people who take diuretics	Dairy products, fish, fruit (especially apricots, bananas, and citrus), legumes, meat, poultry, sea vegetables, sunflower seeds, vegetables (especially potatoes), whole grains
Saponins	Phytonutrients	Lower cholesterol and triglycerides by facilitating their use in cell membrane repair Interact with cholesterol in the stomach and intestines, preventing cholesterol absorption	Alfalfa sprouts, asparagus, beans, chickpeas (garbanzo beans), green beans, green peas, haricot beans, lentils, mung bean shoots, navy beans,

Nutrient	Type	Function	Food Sources
Saponins *(continued)*	Phytonutrients	Promote cholesterol excretion	silverbeet, soybeans, spinach
Selenium	Mineral	Important for elasticity of tissues Keeps blood vessel walls flexible Acts as an antioxidant Should be used together with vitamin E because they potentiate each other and each facilitates the other's absorption	Broccoli, garlic, kidney, liver, meats, mushrooms, seafood, wheat germ, whole grains
Sodium	Mineral	Increases blood pressure in people with hypertension but is important in maintaining fluid balance	Celery, salt
Sulfur	Mineral	Helps in liver detoxification Is especially important for people who take statin drugs, which stress the liver	Broccoli, Brussels sprouts, cabbage, garlic, leeks, mustard, onions
Vanadium	Mineral	Assists with glucose utilization Assists with cholesterol and fat metabolism	Buckwheat, eggs, parsley, soybeans
Vitamin A and beta-carotene	Vitamins	Act as antioxidants	Cheese, eggs, fish liver oils, green and yellow fruits and vegetables, milk, sea vegetables

VITAMIN B-COMPLEX

Before we look at the individual B vitamins, I'd like to make a few general remarks about the B family. Although each of the B vitamins has a different specific purpose in the proper functioning of the body, it is important to realize that the B group works together synergistically and that it works best in conjunction with other vitamins as well. I can't emphasize enough the importance of eating the full array of foods in this vitamin group for general health and specifically for cardiovascular health. If you are elderly, vegan, or alcoholic, studies have shown that you are at greater risk of vitamin deficiencies in these areas, and you will need to be especially vigilant about increasing your consumption of these foods and also using supplements.

Nutrient	Type	Function	Food Sources
Vitamin B_1 (thiamin)	Vitamin	Helps to metabolize micronutrients including carbohydrates, proteins, and fats Helps to ensure that fats do not deposit on arterial walls but are disposed of Is essential for heart muscle function	Arame, brewer's yeast, fish, meat, molasses, nuts, sunflower seeds, whole grains
Vitamin B_2 (riboflavin)	Vitamin	Helps to metabolize proteins, carbohydrates, and fats Builds body tissue and red blood cells	Arame, beef, blackstrap molasses, eggs, fish, hijiki, kombu, leafy green vegetables, legumes, nuts, poultry, whole grains
Vitamin B_3 (niacin)	Vitamin	Regulates platelet clotting Helps to decrease the liver's production of VLDL	Agar, eggs, legumes, meat, nori, nuts, poultry, wakame, whole grains
Vitamin B_5 (pantothenic acid)	Vitamin	Acts as a potent antioxidant Aids in metabolism of proteins, fats, and carbohydrates	All plant and animal products, especially organ meat

Nutrient	Type	Function	Food Sources
Vitamin B_5 (pantothenic acid) *(continued)*	Vitamin	Aids in production of red blood cells Supports the adrenal glands during stress	
Vitamin B_6 (pyridoxine)	Vitamin	Plays a part in digestion and enzyme activity Boosts the immune system Helps to metabolize fatty acids and proteins Maintains low levels of homocysteine	Agar, avocado, bananas, beans (especially soy), dulse, egg yolk, fish, liver, milk, peanuts, peas, poultry, walnuts, whole grains
Vitamin B_{12} (cyano-cobalamin)	Vitamin	Aids in digestion Assists in formation of blood cells Assists in formation of DNA Helps to maintain low homocysteine levels	Agar, dairy products, dulse, eggs, fermented soy products (tempeh, tofu), fish (herring, liver), meat, nutritional yeast, poultry
Folic acid (folate)	Vitamin	Helps with red blood cell formation Helps with production of hemoglobin Helps with production of collagen that makes blood vessel walls elastic Helps in liver's detoxification and anti-inflammatory processes Helps to maintain low homocysteine levels	Beef, bran, chicken liver, green leafy vegetables, lamb, legumes, pork, whole wheat, yeast
Vitamin C	Vitamin	Acts as an antioxidant Helps to lower LDL cholesterol	Berries, broccoli, citrus fruit, green

Nutrient	Type	Function	Food Sources
Vitamin C (continued)	Vitamin	Helps to raise HDL cholesterol Helps to reduce high blood pressure Helps to protect against stroke	vegetables, melons, sea vegetables (agar, dulse, kombu, nori, wakame), tomatoes
Vitamin E	Vitamin	Acts as a blood thinner Acts as an antioxidant	Dark green leafy vegetables, dulse, eggs, legumes, nuts, vegetable oils, wheat germ, whole grains
Vitamin K	Vitamin	Necessary for healthy blood clotting	Beef, green leafy vegetables, liver
Zinc	Mineral	Activates the immune system Protects the liver from chemical damage Promotes wound healing Promotes insulin production	Beans and peas (dried), eggs, legumes, meats, poultry, seafood, soybeans, sunflower seeds, whole grains

The Food Pyramid

Many of us were taught to eat a healthy, well-balanced diet based on the four basic food groups. Today's experts have rejected that concept. Instead, they prefer the model of a food pyramid, developed by the U.S. Department of Agriculture's (USDA's) Center for Nutrition Policy and Promotion and adopted by the U.S. Department of Health and Human Services (HHS). The U.S. government urges all Americans to follow its guidelines.

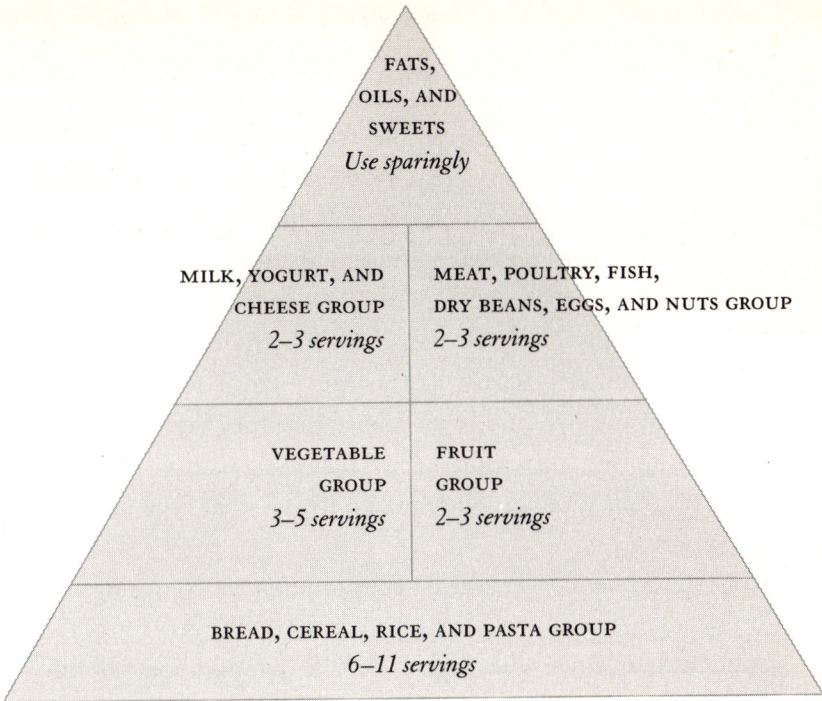

Figure 10.1 The USDA's Food Pyramid

Although the pyramid represents an improvement over the outdated food groups, it is still deficient. Here are some of the things that are wrong with it:

1. Starchy foods form the exclusive base of the pyramid. This places too great an emphasis on grain products as a dietary staple. Studies of societies whose diet consists primarily of vegetables *and* whole grains show that these populations have the lowest incidence of CVD and cancer. Other studies have pointed to the importance of various fish and other seafood products as dietary staples. And we don't need to travel to the Mediterranean to have these findings confirmed. A recent study of health-care workers found that just one additional daily serv-

ing of fruit or vegetables lowered the risk of heart disease by 4 percent.

2. The pyramid does not differentiate between simple and complex carbohydrates. Many people who have dutifully followed the pyramid's recommendations have found that the large quantities of white bread, pasta, and white rice they ate under the pyramid plan have had a negative effect on their health, particularly in such areas as weight and blood sugar. Since white-flour products are simple carbohydrates and are metabolized almost exactly like sweets (which are placed at the top of the pyramid, with advice that they be used "sparingly"), it makes no sense to urge people to eat six to eleven servings of grain products without specifying what type of grain products.

3. The guidelines concerning fat consumption are confusing and misleading. Fats and oils occupy a position at the very top of the pyramid, together with sweets. But the pyramid does not differentiate between unhealthy saturated or hydrogenated fats and the more healthy polyunsaturated and monounsaturated fats.

4. The pyramid does not distinguish between starchy and nonstarchy vegetables but instead lumps all vegetables together in a single category. But starchy vegetables (like potatoes, yams, and corn) and nonstarchy vegetables (like spinach, asparagus, broccoli, and peppers) are actually metabolized quite differently.

5. The current guidelines do not distinguish between fresh fruit and vegetables and canned, frozen, or cooked fruit and vegetables. As we will see later on, there is a great difference in nutritive value.

6. It is not necessary to eat two to three servings of dairy products daily. In fact, too much dairy can be detrimental for reasons that I will discuss later. Some dairy products are fine and enjoyable, but you can get all the nutrients in dairy products (such as protein and calcium) from other sources.

I am not the first physician to express concern about the USDA's food pyramid. Walter Willett, M.D., of Harvard Medical School has published his own version of the food pyramid that is more in accordance with the Mediterranean diet. It emphasizes whole grains and vegetables as well as essential fatty acids. Dr. Willett's food pyramid represents an enormous step in the right direction. I have developed a food pyramid of my own (which is more like Dr. Willett's than the USDA's but also differs from his) based on my own clinical experience and research. This pyramid forms the basis of the CARE diet.

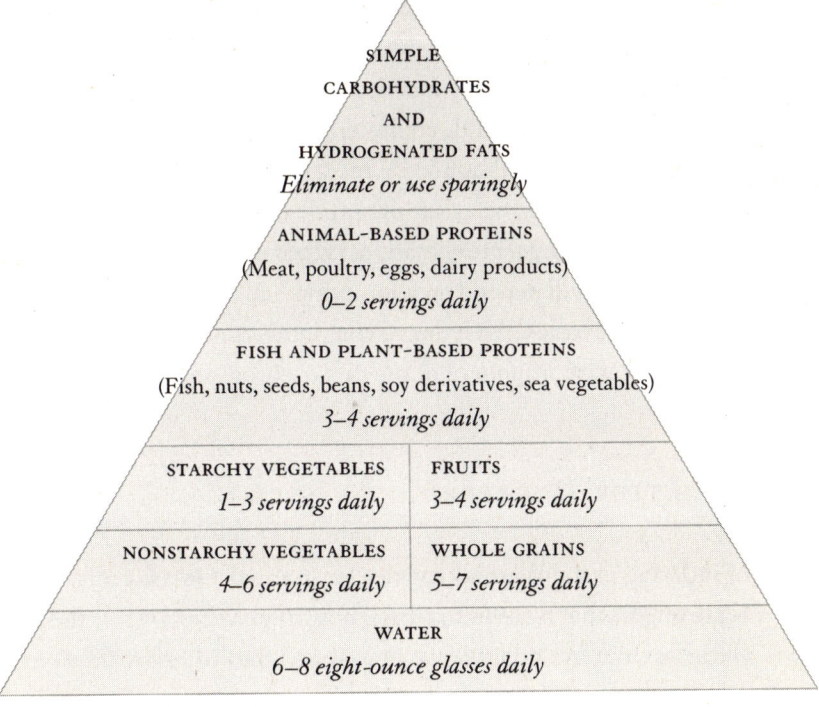

Figure 10.2 The Basic CARE Food Pyramid

Look at figure 10.2. As you can see, the staples of the CARE diet are nonstarchy vegetables and whole grains. Of course, water is an even more fundamental staple; but the bulk of your *food* intake should consist of fresh or very lightly cooked vegetables and whole grains. While the typical American diet generally places protein at the center of the plate, with starch and vegetables as side dishes, vegetables and whole-grain starches should be the central foods, with simpler starches and protein (in that order) as side dishes.

Starchy vegetables and fruits are on the third tier because these are converted by the body into glucose more rapidly than are the second-tier carbohydrates and are lower in fiber.

Protein is divided into two categories. You should try to get most of your protein from fish, dry beans and bean products, soy products, nuts, and seeds, which do not have as much saturated fat as animal products (such as meat, eggs, and dairy products). Moreover, the fat in plant- and fish-based proteins is extremely healthy. Plant-based proteins can lower LDL cholesterol and raise HDL cholesterol, and plants contain fiber and other important nutrients that are absent from animal-based proteins.

For each category in the basic pyramid, I have provided a recommended range of servings. How many servings you personally may have from a given group will depend on your individual degree of risk. We will discuss tailoring the basic CARE diet to your individual needs in chapter 11.

Let's look at each component of my dietary program in greater detail.

PYRAMID TIER 1: WATER

Most of us living in the West take water for granted. Occasionally, we experience droughts that force us to curtail how often we can water the lawn or wash the car, but by and large we can assume that when we turn on the faucet, fresh water will come out. I can't tell you how many of my patients grimace when I urge them to drink more water. They say, "It's boring." They prefer soda, coffee, or other beverages. Studies show that, Americans neglect water, which is so important to healthy functioning, and that, in general, Americans do not have enough fluid intake in their daily diets.

Why do we need water? For starters, 80 percent of our body, by weight, consists of fluid. Our blood is a liquid substance. Sweat, tears, and saliva are all made primarily of water. Our brain floats in cerebrospinal fluid, our joints are lubricated by fluid, our digestive juices are fluid-based, and the mechanisms and apparatus in each cell of our bodies are surrounded by cellular fluid. Although we can derive a certain amount of fluid from our foods, the rest must be taken in liquid form. And while juice, soda, milk, and other drinks are obviously liquids, the body must go through the digestive process in order to extract and use the water in these products. Additionally, fruit juices are sources of concentrated sugar, which is problematic if you are watching your weight or have diabetes. Soda is not only devoid of nutritional value but also often contains harmful chemicals, and sugared sodas contain the highest quantities of sugar in any beverage. One of my colleagues lost ten pounds in two months just by cutting out sugared soft drinks! Water, on the other hand, is chemical- and sugar-free. It also contains no other ingredients for the body to process, so it can immediately be put to use.

Water also serves to flush germs out of the system. This is why it is beneficial to increase your consumption when you are fighting off a cold or some other infection. Water also thins the fluids in your body. When you have a cold, it is better for your mucus to be clear and liquid rather than thick and gluey. You probably know that it is better for your blood to be thinner rather than more viscous. Water softens stool and reduces constipation, and waste matter is disposed of more speedily and efficiently. One of the ways the body disposes of LDL cholesterol is via the stool. The more quickly stools leave the system, the more quickly the LDL cholesterol is removed.

Most professionals agree that you should try to drink the equivalent of eight glasses of water each day. "Equivalent" means that some of this can be taken in the form of juices or other drinks. But you should try to have at least four to six cups in the form of pure water.

Today's tap water often contains impurities—chemicals, heavy metals, toxins, and even, every now and then, parasites. Even boiling does not always remove these. For this reason, I advise all my patients to drink filtered water or spring water from a reputable source. Water filters are quite affordable and easy to find nowadays.

PYRAMID TIER 2: NONSTARCHY VEGETABLES

Some of us spent our childhoods cringing when we heard the word "vegetables." We remember sitting at the dinner table with our mothers, listening to stern lectures about eating our vegetables or we would not be allowed to have dessert or go out and play. We were told that vegetables would make us big and strong. Mother's message was also reinforced by the cartoon character Popeye, whose bulging muscles were attributed to the otherwise despised spinach.

Well, Mom was right. Vegetables are probably the healthiest foods we can eat, not only for our cardiovascular health but also for preventing cancer, building the immune system, and a host of other reasons. Vegetables are packed with all sorts of nutrients. They contain so many wonderful ingredients, in fact, that scientists haven't even discovered or named all of them. These nutrients, often called *phytonutrients* (*phyto* is a Latin root word meaning "plant"), are essential for all areas of health, especially cardiovascular health.

Look again at the list of substances under "Important Nutrients in the Diet" on page 92. Notice how many of them are present in the different types of fruits and nonstarchy vegetables. Each category of vegetable contains different nutrients, although there is some overlap, which is why I encourage my patients to eat a variety of produce culled from a wide range of categories. The basic CARE diet calls for eating four to six servings of nonstarchy vegetables each day (chapter 11 will discuss adjustments to the basic plan, depending on your risk level), but I don't mean that you should just eat lettuce. I believe any diet that focuses exclusively on a single food or food group (such as the grapefruit diet) is unhealthy, even if the food itself is basically a healthy one.

Let's look at several groups of nonstarchy vegetables and review their nutritional content. Please remember that these are just *partial* lists of the wonderfully nutritious contents of vegetables. Scientists simply haven't discovered many of the ingredients in these foods. And remember that there is fiber in all the items listed below.

Cruciferous Vegetables

Examples of this group are broccoli, cauliflower, Brussels sprouts, cabbage, and onions. Cruciferous vegetables contain glutathione, polyphenols, selenium, sulfur, vitamin A, beta-carotene, and vitamin B_5 (pantothenic acid). Broccoli in particular contains vitamin C, carotenoids, and sulfurophane, which is known to have anticarcinogenic properties. Onions contain lots of antioxidants and, like broccoli, contain sulfurophane. These play a particularly central role in detoxifying the liver, which is important for everyone, but especially for anyone who has taken statin drugs.

Broccoli, by the way, is even healthier when it's in the form of sprouts, which are sometimes obtainable at specialty fruit and vegetable stores. These interesting vegetables contain even more antioxidants than mature broccoli and are associated with a variety of health benefits, including protection from cancer and reduction in *Helicobacter pylori,* the virus associated with ulcers and other stomach problems.

Dark Green Vegetables

This group includes kale, collard greens, chard, romaine and other dark green lettuce, spinach, dandelion greens, kohlrabi, endives, Brussels sprouts, parsley, watercress, arugula, and bok choy. Dark green vegetables are good sources of calcium, flavonoids, indoles, iron, para-aminobenzoic acid (PABA), vitamin C, vitamin E, vitamin K, and vitamin B_2 (riboflavin), to name just a few.

Mushrooms

These contain a wide range of B vitamins, as well as chromium and selenium. (Note that while mushrooms are technically fungi, not vegetables, for informal purposes I group them with vegetables because you find them in the fresh produce section of the supermarket.) Until recently, it was thought that mushrooms had no nutritional value. We now know that all mushrooms contain some nutritional value, and three in particular contain important immune-building properties: shiitake, reishi, and maitake. As a culinary aside, you can substitute portabella mushrooms for steak in cooking. They look and taste quite similar to beef but are much better for you.

Summer Squash

Examples here are zucchini and yellow squash. Summer squash contain carotenoids, vitamin A, and folic acid.

Other Vegetables

Following is a list of vegetables not included in the groups above, with short summaries of the wonderful nutrients they contain:

- *Alfalfa sprouts:* calcium, potassium, folic acid, and vitamin A
- *Asparagus:* vitamin A, vitamin C, and beta-carotene
- *Avocado:* copper and vitamin B_6
- *Cauliflower:* copper, calcium, potassium, vitamin C, and vitamin A
- *Celery:* potassium and vitamin A
- *Cucumbers:* potassium, vitamin A, and folic acid
- *Eggplant:* vitamin A
- *Green beans:* saponins
- *Peppers* (green, yellow, orange, and red): flavonoids, vitamin A, and beta-carotene
- *Radishes:* iron
- *Tomatoes:* coumarin, flavonoids, lycopene, vitamin A, and vitamin C

Tips for Preparing and Serving Vegetables

Perhaps you didn't like your vegetables when you were a child because they were not prepared in a very interesting way. Perhaps the spinach looked like an unappetizing mush. (Popeye's certainly did on television.) Vegetables can actually be delicious and interesting to eat. Nibbling on baby carrots, celery slices, or cherry tomatoes is as tasty and pleasant as nibbling on potato chips or pretzel sticks when the urge to snack strikes. Lightly steamed broccoli served with a low-fat sauce is delicious. There are all kinds of ways you can serve vegetables to make them more enjoyable. And because vegetables are so colorful, your plate looks appealing and pretty.

PHYTOSTEROLS: HEART-HEALTHY PHYTONUTRIENTS

Phytosterols are plant-based substances that have been researched since the early 1950s for their cholesterol-lowering effects. Foods containing these compounds have been incorporated into the NCEP-ATP III guidelines for reducing the overall risk of CVD. The FDA has allowed companies that produce products with these compounds to include health claims regarding cardiovascular benefits on their labels. Salad dressings and spreads qualify as "heart-healthy" based on their plant sterol ester content, while dietary supplements in softgel form, snack bars, and spreads qualify on the basis of their plant stanol ester content.

The most common plant sterols that appear in natural forms are called *sitosterol, campesterol,* and *stigmasterol.* When they are saturated (a process that occurs during cooking and heating), they become *plant stanols.* They are similar in molecular structure to cholesterol (note the *sterol* at the end of the word *cholesterol*) but differ in certain aspects of their molecular configuration. The small differences make a big difference in how they are integrated into the body. While cholesterol from animal products is readily absorbed into the body's tissues, phytosterols are poorly absorbed. But they are sufficiently similar to keep the body's cholesterol receptors busy, and they block cholesterol absorption without becoming absorbed themselves. This makes them ideal substitutes for saturated animal fat products (such as butter and lard) and for hydrogenated transfatty acids. They give texture and spreadability to foods without the unhealthy side effects.

A bonus is that they actually lower cholesterol levels! Clinical research has demonstrated that a daily intake of approximately 3 grams of the plant stanol sitostanol reduces total cholesterol by an average of 10 percent and LDL cholesterol by an average of 14 percent. Sitosterol (which is in the *sterol*

(continued)

> rather than the *stanol* form) has also been shown to be effective at lowering cholesterol levels, but larger quantities are needed to produce the same effect. The FDA suggests consuming 1.3 grams of plant sterol esters or 3.4 grams of plant stanol esters daily for cardiovascular benefits.

PYRAMID TIER 2: WHOLE GRAINS

In the CARE food pyramid, whole grains are right above the base of the pyramid as the second most important food category, right next to non-starchy vegetables. Whole grains are associated with a decreased risk of CVD. And they supply complex carbohydrates, giving your body time-released energy over the course of the day. But aside from the fuel that complex carbohydrates offer your body, they also provide you with valuable fiber and nutrients of all sorts.

When I was growing up, many of my friends ate sandwiches on square slices of white bread that looked like sliced cotton wool. Their mothers told them that they should eat the crust because it was "good for them," but they liked the soft inside best and secretly discarded the crust. Now, as an adult and a doctor, I find this interchange somewhat amusing but also very sad. I know now that neither the crust nor the interior of white bread is nutritious, yet millions of American children are still eating the same white-bread sandwiches as steady dietary staples at home and in school. This is due to ignorance and also to economics. Products like white bread are affordable and accessible to thousands of Americans who live below the poverty line. They're also easy to prepare, so working people or harried parents can whip together a meal in minutes.

I urge you to resist the temptation of taking the easy way out and instead to start changing your diet to include more whole grains. Brown rice costs only a little more than white. It is available in fast-cooking formulations, if you don't have the extra time to cook raw brown rice from scratch.

Most legumes, beans, and root vegetables are quite affordable. And you can throw a pot of rice and beans onto the stove at night for dinner the next day, and it can be heated and ready to eat in a matter of minutes. If you have a commitment to your health, you can start to think creatively about convenient ways to substitute complex carbs for simple ones.

The category of whole grains includes brown rice, barley, kasha (buckwheat groats), oats, wheat groats, rye, quinoa, millet, spelt, oat bran, rice bran, and ground flaxseeds. These unrefined grains are packed with an extraordinary number of nutrients, beyond their extra fiber. These include choline, inositol, copper, chromium, iron, magnesium, phosphorus, PABA, selenium, vitamin E, and a variety of B vitamins. Barley and wheat contain lignans, and buckwheat and oats contain vanadium.

I want to make special mention of whole oats because they are one of the best sources of a soluble fiber called *beta-glucan,* which has all sorts of medicinal benefits. To begin with, it lowers cholesterol and protects against CVD.

How do oats help lower cholesterol? It seems that oat bran assists in the excretion of bile acids, which are the acids that the liver forms from cholesterol. The more bile acids are removed from the body, the more the liver must manufacture, and the more cholesterol is removed from the blood to assist in the process. Thus, there is less likelihood of having cholesterol deposited along arterial walls.

It appears, too, that oat bran's effectiveness in excreting bile acids comes from its large beta-glucan content. A similar type of soluble fiber is also found in dried beans and peas. Studies have shown that this is the type of soluble fiber that is most effective in cholesterol-lowering. Interestingly, it also appears to help individuals with diabetes by lowering the amount of insulin they require.

Rice bran has been rising to the foreground of clinical research into bran and whole-grain products. Like oat bran, it has been shown to lower total cholesterol and triglyceride levels by 5 and 15 percent, respectively. A study conducted by Asaf A. Qureshi, Ph.D., and his colleagues in Madison, Wisconsin, found that one out of four subjects with diabetes were able to reduce their daily insulin dosages by adding rice bran to their diet for two months.

Many people who believe that they are eating whole grains are actually eating products that are virtually indistinguishable from those made with white flour. For example, many cereals boast a "high fiber content" or imply that they are "whole grain." You can check out their claims by looking at the ingredients panel on the box. The quantity of fiber is your most important clue to how "whole" a grain product is. Often you end up discovering that your favorite cereal is actually low in dietary fiber and quite high in sugar—even bran cereals that are supposed to provide you with enough fiber to meet your daily requirements. I suggest you avoid any cereal with less than 5 grams of fiber (soluble and insoluble combined) per serving.

While there are exceptions among the commercial cereals, the majority will not meet your dietary fiber requirements. You would be better advised to use brands made of high-quality unrefined grains that are devoid of preservatives and artificial coloring agents and low in refined sugars. Often, these products contain organic ingredients, which means you're not ingesting pesticide residues, either. Some brands I recommend include Arrowhead Mills, Barbara's, Health Valley, Lifestream, and Nature's Path. These are generally healthier and are more likely to contain sufficient quantities of fiber than commercial cereals.

Similarly, commercial "whole-grain breads" are often no better than their white-bread counterparts. If you look at the dietary fiber content you will discover that they, too, are low in fiber and are just paying lip service to the notion of "whole grain." Nutritionist Shari Lieberman, Ph.D., my friend and colleague, sometimes advises her clients to lift a loaf of bread before they buy it. If it's light and airy, you know that it does not contain sufficient quantities of fiber to qualify as a whole-grain product. She tells me that the bread she stocks in her kitchen is almost as heavy as the weights she uses to work out in the gym!

Why is fiber so important? For starters, it adds bulk to your stool, which makes bowel movements more substantial, easier to pass, and more regular. Regular stools do more than simply add to one's comfort level. If waste matter remains in the intestine too long, it begins to rot. If that sounds unpleasant—well, it is. Unexcreted waste serves as a breeding ground for bacteria, which damage the lining of the intestinal tract, hinder the absorption of nutrients, and create a generally toxic environment. Fiber serves as a broom to clean out the intestines. It ensures that waste matter doesn't accumulate along the intestinal walls. This waste includes chemical products that your body should get rid of, such as excess cholesterol.

Fiber disposes of cholesterol and fat before they are absorbed into the system. The fiber "grabs" at cholesterol molecules and attaches them to bile acids produced by the liver, which are designed to break down cholesterol. The fiber, together with its broken-down cholesterol, travels through the intestinal tract and out of the body. That's why a high-fiber diet can reduce total cholesterol and raise HDL levels.

Insoluble fiber does not dissolve in water and remains relatively intact as it passes through your system. Some of its components are lignin, cellulose, and hemicellulose. Soluble fiber, on the other hand, dissolves in water and can be broken down by intestinal bacteria. The pectin and guar gum in soluble fiber, which are by-products of this breakdown, are responsible for the ability of fiber to nab and imprison cholesterol. This is why soluble fiber is so instrumental in lowering cholesterol levels.

The average American diet consists of about 10 to 12 grams of fiber daily. I recommend getting at least 25 grams of fiber, consisting of a combination of both soluble and insoluble fiber.

I believe bread qualifies as a whole-grain product if it contains at least 4 grams of fiber per slice. It is unlikely that you'll find this type of bread in your supermarket. Chances are that you will need to go to a health-food store or, if you are fortunate enough to have one in your area, a natural-foods grocery. Or you can bake your own bread, experimenting with combinations of unbleached white and whole-grain flour until you have come up with a taste, texture, and consistency that satisfy both your culinary and dietary needs.

Here are some other ways to increase your whole-grain consumption:

- Limit your pasta. Even whole-grain pasta (available at health-food stores) is a processed product and therefore less healthy than other forms of whole grains.
- When you eat Chinese food, order brown rice instead of white.
- Sprinkle bran—especially oat bran—onto cereals, mix it into meat loaves and casseroles, and add it to home-baked goods.

It may take some adjustment to incorporate more whole grains into your diet, but it is worth it in the long run.

PYRAMID TIER 3: STARCHY VEGETABLES

Starchy vegetables are an excellent source of complex carbohydrates, though typically they do not contain as much fiber as whole grains. That's why I put them on tier 3—because they should be eaten in moderation, especially by people who have diabetes or who are trying to lose weight. Two notable subcategories of starchy vegetables are root vegetables and winter squash.

Root Vegetables

Root vegetables include beets, carrots, daikon, jicama (Mexican potato), parsnips, potatoes, turnips, sweet potatoes, and yams. These vegetables tend to be starchier than the cruciferous and leafy greens, and qualify as healthy starches for the next category up the food pyramid, but they are still vegetables. Some (notably carrots, sweet potatoes, and yams) are extremely high in vitamin A and beta-carotene. Potatoes have a lot of glutathione and potassium. And those with bright colors are also high in flavonoids.

Winter Squash

Examples of this group are acorn, butternut, pumpkin, and spaghetti squash. Like root vegetables, winter squash is as much a carbohydrate as a vegetable and should be counted as such in your diet. Acorn squash in particular is a source of glutathione.

PYRAMID TIER 3: FRUITS

Fruits are almost as important as vegetables. When your mother put a shiny red apple in your lunch box, she was hoping that you would eat it because it was good for you. Your mother did *not* intend for you to use your apple to bribe your teacher! Again, Mom knew what she was doing; the old adage that an apple a day keeps the doctor away was born from generations of wisdom.

Fruit shares the place of honor with vegetables and whole grains as a significant staple of the CARE diet pyramid, but as with starchy vegetables, it should be eaten more sparingly than nonstarchy vegetables or whole grains. That is because fruit contains a mixture of simple and complex carbohydrates. Eating too much fruit can elevate your blood-sugar levels and add excess weight because you are still consuming a large quantity of simple sugars.

Here are summaries of some of the many varieties of fruits and the wonderful nutrients they contain.

Apples

Apples are one of the best sources of fiber because they contain pectin, which is a soluble fiber. They also contain potassium and vitamin E.

Bananas

Bananas are a wonderful source of magnesium and potassium, a mineral that is especially important for people with high blood pressure. We all know that bananas are great to put into cereal, but they're also wonderful to put into the blender, together with low-fat organic milk or soy milk and berries for a delicious smoothie. And they can be peeled, wrapped in plastic, and frozen. The next day, you have a delicious "Popsicle" for dessert!

Berries

Berries, including strawberries, raspberries, blueberries, blackberries, boysenberries, elderberries, loganberries, and cranberries, are among my favorite foods. I love to eat them, and I love to recommend them to my patients. They're fun to nibble on, sweet and juicy, and have a wide variety of flavors, textures, and colors. They're loaded with vitamin C as well as pectin, and they also contain a wonderful array of flavonoids. (That's what gives them their pretty colors.) They're super high in antioxidants, so they slow the process of LDL oxidation. Additionally, people who eat lots of berries have less sticky blood. So use berries liberally and creatively. Sprinkle them on your cereal, add them to fruit salads and even green salads, or pop them into your mouth when you feel the urge to nibble.

I'd like to make special mention of cranberries and urge you to eat them throughout the year, not only at your Thanksgiving dinners. In pure form, cranberries contain the highest quantity of disease-fighting polyphenols, as compared with nineteen other types of fruit, according to a study conducted by Joe Vinson, Ph.D., a chemist affiliated with the University of Scranton in Pennsylvania.

Remember that phenols help prevent stroke and heart disease, as well as cancer. Additionally, cranberries are quite high in antioxidants and are known to reduce the risk of periodontal disease. It's possible that this is the mechanism through which cranberries confer protective benefits on the cardiovascular system, since gum disorders contribute to CVD. However, it is also possible that the antioxidants in berries fight free radicals and reduce inflammation in the body.

Cranberry juice is known to reduce the unpleasant symptoms of urinary tract infections—perhaps because the antioxidants have an anti-inflammatory effect on the irritated bladder and urethral walls.

The way to obtain maximum benefits from cranberry juice is to drink it raw, although it's very sour. You can mix 1 ounce of juice with water to dilute it. If you find this unbearable, the next best thing is to have fresh or dried cranberries. They are available in supermarkets, like dried raisins. Cranberry sauce is less nutritious than fresh or dried cranberries, but still has some nutrients—especially if you don't overcook it. Lowest on the totem pole is the cranberry juice cocktail products you can buy at the supermarket. These contain only about 27 percent pure juice, and are the least nutritious of all.

I'd also like to mention that strawberries are particularly high in lycopene, an antioxidant also found in tomatoes and watermelons.

Citrus Fruits

The citrus group includes grapefruits, oranges, lemons, limes, tangerines, and clementines. Citrus fruits are high in vitamin C, as most people know. But did you know that citrus fruits also have coumarins, flavonoids, and potassium, and that grapefruits contain glutathione? According to the American College of Cardiology, drinking 2 cups of orange juice per day can result in clinically significant reductions in blood pressure. Daily consumption of orange juice may also result in improved endothelial function.

Figs

Syrup of figs is one of the oldest laxatives (next to prune juice), and with good reason. Fresh figs are loaded with pectin. They're a very tasty and also nutritious treat. One caveat, however: Dried figs, though delicious, are quite high in concentrated sugar and should be eaten only in moderation.

Grapes

Grapes are emerging as one of the most nutritious fruits you can eat. They are extremely high in an antioxidant called *resveratrol* and also high in flavonoids—especially purple grapes and grape products. The flavonoids in grapes are known to improve endothelial function by making the endothelium more elastic. They also have blood-thinning benefits.

Grape juice and red wine contain the same benefits as raw grapes, although they have somewhat less fiber. In a study of twenty-two adults (average age: sixty-four) with documented coronary artery disease, the participants were asked to drink purple grape juice daily for four weeks. At the end of the study period, they showed improvement in their endothelial function, lipid levels, and glucose metabolism. Best of all, there were no negative side effects. The participants experienced no elevation of blood-sugar levels or triglycerides.

Societies that consume red wine on a regular basis also have a lower incidence of cardiovascular disease. That's because red wine, like purple grape juice, contains a polyphenol that is known to inhibit endothelin-1, a protein that constricts blood vessels. But don't get carried away! Limit your intake of wine to three glasses a week. All alcohol places an enormous burden on the liver, and excessive quantities have an adverse effect on all sorts of bodily functions, including cholesterol metabolism, blood pressure, and sugar metabolism. Alcohol is also known to contribute to obesity.

Finally, I want to emphasize that when you drink grape juice or wine, you should try to get organic products because grapes are notoriously high in pesticide residue levels, especially if they are imported. Try also to get wine and grape juice that are free of *sulfites,* which are chemicals that have been associated with cancer as well as severe allergic reactions—especially among people who have asthma.

Pomegranates

New research conducted by an Israeli scientist named Dr. Michael Aviram shows that pomegranates can help increase blood levels of an enzyme called *paraoxonase,* which appears to be important in helping to break up arterial plaque. Dr. Aviram's studies indicate that drinking just 4 ounces of pomegranate juice a day helps to reduce arterial lesions.

Other Fruits

Following is a list of fruits not included in the groups above, with short summaries of the wonderful nutrients they contain:

- *Mango:* potassium and vitamin A
- *Melons* (cantaloupe, honeydew): vitamin A, potassium, and vitamin C

- *Pears:* very high levels of pectin
- *Pineapple:* very high levels of potassium, vitamin A, and vitamin C
- *Pitted fruits* (peaches, plums, nectarines, and cherries): potassium and vitamin A
- *Watermelon:* high levels of flavonoids and antioxidants (especially lycopene) as well as fiber

Tips for Preparing and Serving Fruit

Like the nonstarchy vegetables we discussed above, fruits should be eaten raw as often as possible. You can bite into them, cut them up on a plate, make a fruit salad, or purée them into a smoothie. They retain the maximum nutritional value that way. Like vegetables, fruits lose their nutritional content if they are left standing out too long.

Fruit juices are highly nutritious, but not as nutritious as the whole product because they lack the pulp, which contains fiber. Juice is metabolized more quickly than whole fruit, because the body does not have to separate fiber from juice, eliminate the fiber, and absorb the juice. For this reason, juice is metabolized as a simple rather than a complex carbohydrate. You need to watch your fruit-juice intake even more carefully than your fruit.

Cooked and canned fruit have more fiber than fruit juice, but the fiber has been softened and much of the nutritional content leached out. Eating cooked fruit is better than eating no fruit, but fresh fruit is best. If you must cook your fruit, the best way of doing so is not by boiling or steaming but by baking. Baked apples (with some raisins and cinnamon) are a delicious dessert, as are baked pears.

PYRAMID TIER 4: FISH AND PLANT-BASED PROTEINS

Protein is an essential part of your diet because it contains amino acids. These are crucial building blocks of health, indispensable for your muscles, bones, skin, and hormones, and for neurotransmitters. Some dietary amino acids are called *essential* because your body cannot manufacture them independently. It relies on the food you eat for the raw materials to make amino acids into protein. Protein foods should account for 20 percent of your daily calories. This means three to four servings daily.

Most people are aware that they need protein in their diets, but they associate protein primarily with meat, poultry, dairy products, and eggs. They do not realize that many plant products contain as much protein as animal-based products, and are also much healthier.

The CARE diet gives fish and plant sources of protein priority over animal sources. That's because plant-based proteins *don't* have the high quantities of saturated fat and cholesterol present in animal-based proteins and because plant-based proteins *do* have an array of other wonderful nutrients that are absent from animal-based protein foods. Fish also contain more nutrients and less fat than proteins derived from other animal sources.

Let's look at the extraordinary array of fish and plant-based protein foods available. (Note: Lest there be any doubt, I am well aware that fish are not vegetables and, indeed, are a class of animal. But I have combined fish and plant-based proteins in a single category in my food pyramid because both are good protein sources. When I speak of animal-based proteins, you should understand the term to refer to land animals rather than sea creatures.)

Fish

All fish contains protein. In fact, it is one of the most concentrated sources of protein you can get. But fish has a lot more going for it than merely its protein content. Fish—especially cold-water fish such as salmon, cod, mackerel, sea bass, halibut, sardines, and anchovies—is very high in omega-3 EFAs, specifically eicosapentaenoic acid (EPA) and docosahexaenoic acid (DHA). Protein and EFAs are not the only nutritious elements found in fish. Most fish also contain biotin (especially sardines), magnesium, phosphorus, selenium, vitamin A and beta-carotene, vitamin B_{12} (especially herring and mackerel), folic acid, and vitamin B_2.

Theoretically, we should be able to eat fish in lavish quantities. Unfortunately, however, environmental pollution has affected the safety of our fish. The oceans are filled with mercury and other heavy metals, which find their way into the tissue of the fish we eat. Ingesting large quantities of mercury and heavy metals can be toxic. It actually increases the risk of CVD by leading to congestive heart failure and arrhythmias and contributing to the proliferation of free radicals. In general, the types of fish and seafood that are relatively low in mercury include salmon (fresh and canned), shrimp, flounder, and halibut. At the other end of the scale, those generally highest in mercury content include shark, swordfish, king mackerel, and tilefish. Pike, bass, walleye, and muskie tend to fall somewhere in between, with moderate levels of mercury.

My best advice to you is to try to get your fish from organic fish farms whenever possible. These fish have far lower concentrations of mercury and other heavy metals than their ocean-bred counterparts. Farm-raised fish are available in many health-food stores and some supermarkets. You can also limit your consumption of fish to three times a week and rely more heavily on plant-based protein sources.

Nuts

Nuts such as almonds, cashews, pecans, pine nuts, pistachios, hazelnuts (filberts), walnuts, and macadamia nuts are among the best sources of protein and are also excellent sources of monounsaturated fatty acids. Nuts—especially walnuts, almonds, and pecans—are high in polyphenols, which inhibit the oxidation of LDL cholesterol, a step in the development of arterial plaque. Nuts are also high in fiber, calcium, copper, coumarins, magnesium, phosphorus, vitamin E, and several of the B vitamins.

Studies have found that people who eat nuts regularly have a lower incidence of heart attack as compared with people who rarely or never eat them. Similarly, one study found that participants who ate 28 grams (nearly 1 ounce) of walnuts three times a day for four weeks experienced an average 12 percent reduction in total cholesterol and an 18 percent reduction in LDL cholesterol. Similar findings have emerged concerning other nuts, such as almonds, cashews, pecans, macadamia nuts, and pistachios. In fact, I like to call these the *super six*. If you are going to incorporate nuts into your diet, these are the ones I recommend. You can sprinkle them on salads or nibble on them raw. Many health-food stores carry cashew and almond butter, which make excellent alternatives to peanut butter for sandwiches.

A note about peanuts and peanut butter: Although peanuts are high in protein, I generally do not recommend them. Technically, by the way, they are legumes, not nuts, but that's not the problem with them; as you know, I recommend many legumes for their nutritious qualities. But peanuts contain a compound called *aflatoxin*. This is a mold that is not only associated with allergies in children—peanuts are decidedly more allergenic than other nuts—but also may be associated with an increased risk of liver cancer. So I recommend other nut butters, such as cashew or almond butter, for your children's (and your) sandwiches.

If you are trying to lose weight, you should eat nuts in moderation. Even though the fat they contain is healthy fat, it still makes them high in calories.

Seeds

Edible seeds include sunflower seeds, flaxseeds, sesame seeds, and pumpkin seeds. Seeds are also high in protein and contain nutritious monounsaturated fats. Here are some of the other nutrients they contain: lignan, phosphorus, potassium (especially sunflower seeds), vitamin B_1, and zinc (especially sunflower seeds).

Add seeds to salads, sandwiches (they lend a wonderful extra crunch), and stews for a lively and unusual surprise. But beware the trail mixes sold in the so-called natural-foods sections of supermarkets or even health-food stores. They usually contain raisins and other dried fruits, which are concentrated sources of simple carbohydrates. Many also have chemical preservatives such as sulfites added to keep the dried fruits colorful and soft. Sulfites might be carcinogenic and have also been associated with allergic reactions and asthma. It is better for you to assemble your own trail mix, consisting of unsweetened nuts and seeds, with just a few dried raisins and cranberries, unsulfured if you can get them.

Legumes

Examples of legumes include split peas, peanuts, soybeans, chickpeas (garbanzo beans), lentils, and beans. Legumes—especially beans—are good sources of protein, as well as of complex carbohydrates.

Legumes are packed with so many nutrients, it's hard to know where to start. I'd like to list them individually, since they have an array of wonderful phytochemicals, some individual and some overlapping. They are also high in iron and provide an alternative to red meat as a source of this mineral. But iron isn't the only mineral in beans and legumes. They also contain calcium, magnesium, potassium, and phosphorus. Finally, all legumes are rich in the B vitamins, especially vitamin B_2, vitamin B_3, and folic acid. And they have lots of fiber, too, approximately 6 to 8 grams per cup.

Following is a list of beans and legumes with short summaries of the nutrients they contain:

- *Beans* (aduki, black, kidney, mung, fava, lima, navy, and others, as well as black-eyed peas and chickpeas): copper, coumarins, magnesium, phosphorus, saponins, protein, and vitamin B_6
- *Lentils:* saponins and protein
- *Soybeans:* biotin, choline, inositol, phosphorus, saponins, vanadium, and vitamin B_6; soybeans (and, incidentally, chickpeas) are also high in *phytoestrogens,* which can be important sources of natural estrogen replacement for menopausal and postmenopausal women
- *Peas:* copper, magnesium, phosphorus, and vitamin B_6
- *Peanuts:* chromium, protein, vitamin B_6, and calcium (I don't recommend eating large quantities—remember, peanuts contain aflatoxin and are highly allergenic—but in small quantities, peanuts are nutritious)

Sea Vegetables

It may surprise you to learn that the ocean yields not only fish but also sea vegetables. When we encounter them at the beach, we call them seaweed and consider them a nuisance. But some societies (such as the Japanese) and some populations within American society (such as those who eat macrobiotic diets) emphasize sea vegetables as dietary staples. Most Americans encounter them most commonly in sushi, but there is an abundance of other uses for them. These products are extremely high in protein and minerals, and make excellent and wonderfully nutritious alternatives to the run-of-the mill protein foods found on most American tables.

The health benefits of sea vegetables are enormous. For starters, they contain a great deal of fiber. They actually dissolve fat, making them quite useful for those seeking to reduce cholesterol levels. Additionally, they improve skin tone, prevent wrinkles, improve hair quality, and neutralize radioactive materials.

Following is a list of sea vegetables and the nutrients they contain, as well as a few words on how you can use them in your diet.

- *Agar:* fiber; vitamins A, B_1, B_6, B_{12}, C, D, and K; and biotin. Agar has a gel-like effect. It can be purchased either in tightly wrapped bars or in flake form. It has virtually no calories. It also has no taste, which means it can blend into anything you're cooking. Use agar for making natural fruit jello or jam (you can add unsweetened fruit juice) or any other item with a gel-like consistency. One tablespoon of agar flakes will cause one cup of liquid to gel, while one bar will have that effect on up to three cups of liquid. If you're in a hurry, you can use the flakes, which can cause boiling liquid to gel within two to three minutes (stir occasionally). Bars take longer—you need to break them into pieces and add them to cool liquid, then boil for fifteen minutes.
- *Arame:* protein, potassium, iron, calcium, iodine, phosphorus, and vitamins A, B_1, and B_2. After being harvested, arame is cooked, then sun-dried. The product you buy will look like

short black strands. It needs to be reconstituted prior to use. Soak for about five minutes in warm water before adding it to your recipe. Use it in your favorite spaghetti sauce, and in soups (especially hot and sour, vegetable, and noodle soups).
- *Dulse:* iron, protein, calcium, phosphorus, iodine, potassium, magnesium, and vitamins A, C, B_6, B_{12}, and E. There are all kinds of interesting ways to use this versatile product. It can be used as a snack food, straight out of the package, or it can be toasted or reconstituted. Its tangy, salty flavor makes it great for dipping into yogurt or dressing as an alternative to crackers or chips. It can also be used as a substitute for bacon in a "BLT" sandwich. To do this, toast the dulse in a moderately hot, dry skillet until it becomes dull brownish-green. The toasted dulse can be crumbled over salad or used in other dishes as well.
- *Hijiki:* calcium, phosphorus, iron, protein, and vitamins A and B_2. For people unaccustomed to its strong ocean flavor, it can be hard to learn to like hijiki. But it's worth acquiring a taste for this incredibly nutritious product. One tablespoon of hijiki provides fourteen times more calcium than a cup of milk. Hijiki is usually sold in packages of small dark, curly pieces. Reconstituted, it will expand to four times its volume. Soak it in warm water for ten to fifteen minutes, then add a small quantity as a garnish for a hot grain or noodle dish.
- *Kombu* and *kelp:* iron, calcium, phosphorus, and vitamins A, B_2, and C. These sea vegetables have similar flavors and usages. They are usually dark olive green in color and are packaged in wide flat pieces. You can reconstitute by cutting into four- to five-inch strips, then soaking in water for five to ten minutes. Add small strips or squares to stir-fry vegetables, stews, soups, or hot grain dishes. You may also find it tasty to add noodles flavored with miso or soy sauce.
- *Nori:* calcium, iron, potassium, magnesium, phosphorus, iodine, and vitamins A, B_2, B_3, C, and D, and niacin. Nori is the black, paper-thin cover used to wrap sushi. It comes in large cel-

lophane packages and looks like dark purplish or olive brown sheets. But don't try to reconstitute it. Instead, you should toast it before using it as a wrap for rice, sushi, or other products. It turns these healthful products (to which you can add tofu, cucumber, or other vegetables) into easy-to-eat finger foods that are higher in nutritional content than almost any other snack food. Aside from its impressive protein content (35 percent), nori contains as much vitamin A as carrots.

- *Wakame:* iron, calcium, magnesium, phosphorus, and vitamins C, A, B_2, and B_{12}. This sea vegetable has a much milder flavor than kombu, but is used similarly. It comes in long strands, approximately two inches wide. To reconstitute, simply tear off the desired amount and soak in warm water for ten minutes. It will expand to two to three times its volume. Try adding a small amount of chopped reconstituted wakame and scallions to scrambled eggs or split pea or miso soup. This will potentiate your meal by increasing your intake of calcium, phosphorus, and iron.

PYRAMID TIER 5: ANIMAL-BASED PROTEINS

I group meat, poultry, dairy products, and eggs together because all of them are high in protein, but all of them also contain saturated fat. But unless you are a vegan (a person who consumes no foods of animal origin) and choose to avoid these products for humanitarian reasons, I encourage you to continue incorporating them into your diet—but on a limited basis. All of these foods contain important nutrients, but they should not be the mainstay of each meal.

A few general remarks before we look at specific products.

I advise my patients to obtain organically raised meat, poultry, dairy, and eggs whenever possible. There are several reasons for this. Most livestock are routinely given antibiotics to prevent infection. You might think that this is done for the sake of the consumer, but it is actually done for the sake of the farmer. It is inconvenient and expensive for a farmer to treat a sick animal and certainly to treat massive outbreaks of infectious diseases. It's easier to administer an antibiotic as a preventive. The trouble is that these antibiotics enter the meat, poultry, milk, and eggs that we eat. This means that we are ingesting antibiotics that are unnecessary and even counterproductive to human health.

Animals are also fed growth hormones to speed weight gain. This is definitely for the sake of the farmer. The larger and more quickly the animal grows, the more money it brings in! Again, these growth hormones are detrimental to human beings. They have been associated with unnaturally early puberty in certain populations, and some studies have suggested an association with breast cancer as well.

Finally, pesticide residues in animal feed can be transmitted to the consumer—especially in organ meats, such as the kidney and liver. I advise my patients to avoid those foods completely or to eat them sparingly.

I recommend organic foods from a humanitarian point of view also. Generally speaking, farmers who use alternative means of feeding and caring for animals also are more humane. For example, I advise my patients to purchase only free-range poultry, which is allowed to move around the coop rather than being compressed into tiny cages. This has not only spiritual but also health-related benefits. Animals that are allowed to move freely have more muscle and less fat. (For this reason, wild game makes an excellent low-fat alternative to cattle for those who enjoy eating meat.) And of course, organic farming is much safer for the environment as a whole.

Now let's look at individual food categories within this group.

Meat

Red meat is extremely high in nutrients such as chromium, iron, phosphorus, vitamins B_1, B_3, B_{12}, and zinc. Lamb and pork are good sources of folic acid.

To minimize the fat content of your meat, trim all excess fat off before you cook it. Grill and broil meats instead of frying, roasting, or baking them. That way, larger quantities of fat will drain off. And watch out for those commercially prepared hamburgers, cold cuts, and hot dogs. They usually contain the lowest quality and highest fat components of the meat. Often, they also contain chemical additives.

Poultry

What would Thanksgiving be without a turkey? And what would your mother bring over when you have the flu, if not chicken soup? Poultry is an integral part of the diet of most Americans. I certainly prefer poultry to red meat, because chicken and turkey breast are usually leaner than red-meat products. Poultry also has different nutrients than meat products, although there is some overlap. Poultry contains iron, phosphorus, vitamins B_2, B_6, folic acid (in chicken liver), and zinc.

When preparing poultry, be sure to remove the skin and as much of the fat as possible. Although chicken and turkey are often cooked within the skin so as to ensure a moister, more succulent outcome, the moist texture is due to the heavy fat content and should be avoided. You can moisten chicken in many other ways. You can brush your poultry with any number of interesting liquids or pastes to serve your taste, then cover and bake. For example, you can use a mixture of canola oil, a little honey, and fruit juice for a sweet-and-sour taste, or tomato paste for a hearty effect. Cutting up vegetables such as onions, which express a great deal of fluid as they cook, is another way to add moisture. Chicken can be grilled as well as roasted or baked. It can be cubed and skewered, together with pieces of pepper, tomato, and onion, to make shish kebob.

A word about chicken soup, which is often very high in fat: When you make chicken soup, allow it to cool before serving. The fat will rise to the surface and congeal, making it easy to skim off. You will find you are lifting a hardened substance rather than skimming a liquid. If you must avoid all saturated fats completely, use chicken cutlets instead of whole chicken parts. There is virtually no fat in these. To add flavor and color, you can purée a few carrots and throw in soup greens and onions.

Dairy Products

Dairy products are a staple of most American diets. However, unless you use nonfat varieties, dairy products contain saturated fat. Moreover, I would caution you against such products as nonfat cottage cheese, which gets its creamy texture from chemical additives. I would rather see you have the small quantity of fat in low-fat cottage cheese than put chemical products into your body.

I also caution you against the use of non-organic dairy products. The cows are fed antibiotics and growth hormones and graze on grass that has been treated with pesticides. If you are eating dairy, I urge you to use only organic products, which are now widely available in supermarkets and health-food stores.

The American Dairy Council has touted the high calcium content of milk with good reason. Additional nutrients in dairy products are biotin (found in milk), chromium (cheese), phosphorus, vitamin A and beta-carotene, and vitamins B_6 and B_{12}.

A caveat about calcium and dairy products: Many people do not tolerate dairy foods well, whether due to allergy, lactose intolerance, or personal preference. Refer again to "Important Nutrients in the Diet" on page 92, which lists other foods that contain calcium.

Eggs

A book about cholesterol and heart disease that does not have a thorough discussion of the notorious egg would be deficient indeed. Most Americans reflexively think of eliminating eggs when they hear the words *cholesterol reduction*. Eggs certainly have gotten bad press, and they do contain approximately 200 milligrams of cholesterol per yolk. But eggs are not all bad, and if you eat them in moderation, they can be nutritious and enjoyable, especially if you follow the other heart-healthy practices recommended in this book. And I would rather see you eat a good, old-fashioned wholesome egg than a chemical egg substitute.

Egg whites are high in protein and can be eaten in large quantities without any concern about the fat content. But you don't have to completely eliminate egg yolks from your diet. They contain important nutrients, such as biotin, choline and inositol, phosphorus, PABA, vanadium, vitamin A and beta-carotene, vitamin E, zinc, and vitamins B_2, B_3, B_6, and B_{12}. They also contain naturally occurring lecithin, which helps to metabolize the cholesterol.

PYRAMID TIER 6: SIMPLE CARBOHYDRATES AND HYDROGENATED FATS

I have put refined flour products, which the USDA groups together with grains at the base of its pyramid, at the very top. The USDA pyramid may not distinguish between refined and whole grains, but I consider white bread, bagels, and pasta to be as detrimental as table sugar and honey. If you start to regard sugar and white-flour products as very unusual treats reserved for rare, special occasions, you will be taking an important step toward good health.

I would *like* to say that no one should ever eat any of these items, but I know that's not realistic. In my twenty years of clinical experience, I have learned that most people simply will not adhere strictly to a diet that prohibits their favorite foods. I have therefore come to the conclusion that it is better to build a certain number of splurges into a diet because people who feel they cannot abstain are likely to become discouraged and give up the diet altogether. Please understand that this is not an endorsement of sugar or white-flour products, simply a concession to the realities of human nature.

An important caveat: By splurging, I don't mean overindulging or binging or gorging. One of my patients was on a weight-loss diet. Every time she went "off her diet," she ended up with an "all is lost, so what the heck" attitude. She would stuff herself, then feel guilty. Another patient used to talk about his "cheating days." Once a week, he veered from his cholesterol-lowering regimen to cheat. But instead of limiting himself to one piece of cake or one cheeseburger, he ate all the wrong foods for a whole day, then assiduously stuck to his diet the other six days of the week.

When I say it's okay to splurge, I mean that you can have one piece of cake or one scoop of ice cream. Or you can have one serving of fries, or whatever suits your fancy. Moderation does not seem to be part of the American vocabulary; portion sizes are growing larger, and Americans are also growing larger. It's hard to learn self-limitation, but successful splurging involves incorporating forbidden foods into one's lifestyle in a careful and controlled fashion—*occasionally,* and in small quantities. In my experience, it is the daily assault upon the system of such foods as the morning bowl of cereal with sugar or the white-bread sandwich at lunch that really causes the destruction.

Hydrogenated Fats and Cholesterol: Fact and Myth

There has been a great deal of controversy and confusion regarding fat and cholesterol, and it's worth clarifying what the most recent scientific thinking is. First of all, *all fats are not bad!* Some fat is needed to maintain good health. The majority of your brain and liver is composed of fat. Fats are required for the absorption of the fat-soluble vitamins A, D, E, and K. The key lies in the *type* and *quantity* of each type of fat.

There are basically three types of fats: saturated, polyunsaturated, and monounsaturated fat. The difference between them is found at a molecular level and concerns the configuration of carbon molecules and the number of double bonds between them.

SATURATED FAT

Saturated fat is found primarily—indeed, almost exclusively—in animal products: meat, chicken, dairy products, and eggs, although there are a few fruits and vegetables that have saturated fat, most notably coconut and avocado. The body converts saturated fat into cholesterol. It is therefore the least desirable type of all the fats, since excess cholesterol contributes directly to plaque buildup in the arteries. However, in small quantities, it is not harmful—unless you are on an aggressive cholesterol-lowering diet, which we will discuss in the next chapters. And meat, poultry, and dairy products contain other beneficial substances, such as protein, calcium, and vitamin B_{12}. Even the much-maligned egg yolk has been found to contain helpful nutrients, such as biotin, choline, inositol, phosphorus, para-aminobenzoic acid (PABA), vanadium, vitamin A, beta-carotene, vitamin E, vitamins B_2, B_3, B_6, and B_{12}, and zinc.

POLYUNSATURATED FAT

Polyunsaturated fats are found primarily in nuts and seeds and oils pressed from them, such as sunflower, safflower, almond, walnut, corn, and sesame seed oils. Your body actually needs a certain amount of these oils and the fatty acids found within them. The key is *balance*—too much polyunsaturated fat provides your body with only one type of necessary fat, and this overwhelms certain chemical processes. When cholesterol-conscious Americans began eliminating saturated fats from their diets, they increased their consumption of polyunsaturated fats, which were supposedly cholesterol-free. This created some significant imbalances in fat metabolism.

One additional caveat about polyunsaturated oils: Because they have a more favorable cholesterol profile than saturated oils, doctors started urging their patients to switch from butter to margarine. People were encouraged to reduce their consumption of red meats and cheeses and to increase their consumption of grain products, like crackers and pretzels. What these well-intentioned physicians did not realize was that the processing of vegetable oil into margarine and the type of oil used in commercial crackers may be more detrimental to the body than butter, though for a different reason.

MONOUNSATURATED FAT

The final basic category of fat is called *monounsaturated*. Olive and canola oils fall into this category. These are probably the best for your health.

ESSENTIAL FATTY ACIDS

Some fat is essential to your health. I use the word *essential* here in two ways. One is the common sense of the word, as something that is necessary, even indispensable. But I also use the word in its technical sense. To scientists, an *essential* substance is something that the human body cannot manufacture from other components but that must be imported from outside—taken in through the diet.

As amino acids are the building blocks of proteins, essential fatty acids (EFAs) are the building blocks of fats and oils. Scientists began researching EFAs in earnest when they noticed something striking and strange: Despite consuming large quantities of high-fat whale meat, Eskimo populations did not seem to suffer from cardiovascular disease (and from several other disorders as well) at anywhere near the rate that other people did. Studies that compared Eskimos to Danes, whose diet contained a much lower fat intake, showed that the Danes nevertheless had a much higher incidence of CVD. Clearly, fat was not necessarily such an evil.

Such results have been replicated dozens of times. Researchers have noted a lower incidence of sudden cardiac death among those who regularly consume nuts—a high-fat food—as compared with those who do not eat nuts at all. Interestingly, the Mediterranean diet, which is well known to be associated with a comparatively low incidence of heart disease, is rich not only in fish but also in nuts.

There are two important groups of EFAs. They are called *omega-3* and *omega-6,* designations that are based on their molecular structures. It is important to eat both types of fat, and in the correct proportions, because each has a different function in the body.

The omega-3 fatty acids, which are found in cold-water fish, seafood, flaxseeds, and some leafy green plants, contain several important ingredients with complicated-sounding names. Of particular note are eicosapentaenoic acid (EPA), docosahexaenoic acid (DHA), and alpha-linolenic acid (ALA). One of the most important functions of these chemicals is to fight inflammation in the body. They also stabilize irregularities in heart rhythm and help reduce the stickiness of blood.

The omega-6 family of fatty acids also has important components. Of note is gamma-linolenic acid (GLA), which is highly therapeutic. It is found in certain plants, such as borage, evening primrose, and black currants. It is the healthiest of all the omega-6 fatty acids, which serve to balance the omega-3 group. The body uses essential fatty acids to produce important substances known as *prostaglandins,* which are similar to hormones and regulate bodily functions, including the inflammatory response. Some prostaglandins have the effect of promoting inflammation, while others inhibit it. With the correct balance of available EFAs, the body knows when to produce pro-inflammatory prostaglandins and when to produce anti-inflammatory prostaglandins.

Most people in Western societies ingest more omega-6 fatty acids than they need, and proportionally less omega-3. Increasing your omega-3 intake is one of the greatest gifts you can give your health because it will correct the omega-3 to omega-6 balance. Scientists have demonstrated that people who ingest just 0.6 to 2.4 grams (600 to 2,400 milligrams) of omega-3 EFAs per week have a 20 percent lower than average risk of mortality from all causes, including cardiovascular disease, cancer, immune disorders, and infectious diseases. Interestingly, the use of statin drugs yields a 29 percent reduction in mortality as well. But EFAs do not have the built-in risks and negative side effects associated with statin drugs. What amazes me is that if the omega-3 EFAs were a new drug of some sort, every pharmaceutical company in the country would be competing to develop them and clamoring for approval from the FDA. And in fact, in February 2002, the FDA approved the following statement to appear on the label of omega-3 fatty acid dietary supplements: "Consumption of omega-3 fatty acids may reduce the risk of coronary heart disease." Foods high in omega-3 fatty acids include fish (especially mackerel, Atlantic herring, albacore tuna, Chinook salmon, anchovies, Coho salmon, Greenland halibut, rainbow trout, and Atlantic cod, which contain primarily DHA and EPA), nuts and seeds (especially almonds, flaxseeds, and walnuts), green leafy vegetables (such as spinach, Brussels sprouts, and kale), olive oil, raw soybeans, leeks, pinto beans, purslane, and wheat germ. Fish primarily contain DHA and EPA; plant foods contain primarily ALA.

HYDROGENATED FAT

To turn liquid oil into margarine, a process called *hydrogenation* must occur. This alters the structure of the original oil by adding extra hydrogen atoms so the oil hardens into a spreadable, butterlike substance at room temperature. The new type of fat, called *transfatty acid* (TFA), is found in most commercially baked products, as well as in margarine and vegetable shortening. Hydrogenation also occurs in fats that are heated to very high temperatures repeatedly, like the oils used in fast-food restaurants to deep-fry potatoes.

TFA is not a naturally occurring substance. It is not recognized by the body, and in order to try to metabolize TFAs, enzymes ordinarily used to digest other foods are "kidnapped" and given a new job: to try to make heads or tails of this strange material and break it down into a form usable by the body. The result is that many enzymatic steps that are essential to healthy digestion are blocked, the normal metabolism of normal fats is inhibited, and the body is robbed of essential fatty acids necessary for all sorts of bodily functions.

TFAs gum up not only the enzymatic pathways but also the pathways your body uses to detoxify. This means that your body is so busy trying to get rid of these bizarre molecules that it neglects the cholesterol molecules, which build up in the bloodstream and contribute to plaque.

And TFAs are notorious contributors to the spread of free radicals in the system. They cause a free-radical rampage that overwhelms your body's ability to dispose of these destructive agents.

The potential danger caused by TFAs is so significant that the FDA is considering requiring a warning label on food products indicating how much hydrogenated oil they contain. This is a step in the right direction, but America actually lags behind other countries in TFA consciousness. In Europe, for example, most foods are allowed to contain no more than 1 percent hydrogenated oils. In the United States, by contrast, a product such as vegetable shortening consists of 40 percent hydrogenated fat!

It is estimated that TFAs account for up to 60 percent of the fat in many processed foods. The average American's intake is between 10 and 20 grams of TFA per day. Since there is no safe dose of these destructive substances and they have no known health benefits, it would be best for you to keep your own intake as close to zero as possible. In fact, it's been estimated that TFAs may contribute to as many as 30,000 CVD deaths each year.

So I am not an advocate of margarine as a substitute for butter. In my opinion, it is better to have a small pat of butter than to lavishly smear your cracker (undoubtedly made with hydrogenated oil itself) with margarine. Better yet, use olive oil as a dip for your bread and sprinkle some fresh pepper on for taste. As you will see, you can occasionally indulge in butter, and even in ice cream, if you keep your intake within modest limits and otherwise engage in a heart-healthy lifestyle.

Off the Pyramid: Additional Beneficial Foods

I have a few favorite foods I like to recommend for my patients to enjoy. They are not included in the basic pyramid guidelines, but they are wonderful and will benefit your palate as well as your health.

GINGER

Although you can obtain ginger as an herb, I recommend it for use as a component of your diet. First of all, it's delicious. It is wonderful in baked goods or even in salads for a fascinating zingy flavor. You can get it dried in small cubes, which are a wonderful substitute for candy. Ginger has anti-inflammatory properties. Studies have shown that it is effective in lowering CRP levels, and, of course, it battles the inflammatory process that goes on in your blood vessels. Ginger also inhibits platelet formation, leading to thinner blood.

TEA

Solid evidence is mounting that drinking tea can prevent the type of cell damage that can lead to cancer, heart disease, and perhaps other illnesses as well. According to scientists who spoke at a meeting sponsored by the USDA, the Tea Council, and the American Cancer Society, it may soon be time to add tea to the list of fruits and vegetables that experts urge Americans to eat as often as possible.

How is tea beneficial? It appears that tea contains a large quantity of a flavonoid called *elagic acid,* which helps prevent platelet stickiness. And green tea in particular lowers total cholesterol levels and reduces the risk of contracting all forms of cancer, especially breast cancer. It significantly inhibits the oxidation of LDL cholesterol and also improves endothelial function. If you don't like tea, you can obtain green tea as a dietary supplement in capsule or extract form.

Putting It Together

You now know the building blocks of the CARE food pyramid, but you may be wondering how to put it all together. How large is a serving?

How do I know how many to eat? How many treats and liberties can I have? What if I'm trying to lose weight? What if I'm a vegetarian? What if my cholesterol levels are normal but my homocysteine level is too high? Or my LDL cholesterol is too high but everything else is normal? And how do I know whether to count chickpeas as a protein or a complex carbohydrate, or whether I should have dairy or soy for dinner?

The next chapter will answer these and similar questions and will help you tailor a diet to your individual needs in a way that takes account of your risk-factor profile, lifestyle, and personal preferences.

11 Customizing the CARE Diet

Animals feed themselves, men eat; but only wise men know the art of eating.
— Anthelme Brillat-Savarin

It's good for everyone to be acquainted with the basic plan. And if your risk level is low (level 1), you can follow the basic guidelines outlined in the previous chapter. But if your risk level is higher, this chapter will help you fine-tune the components of the CARE diet program to suit your individual needs.

Level 2: Mild Risk

Figure 11.1 illustrates the proportions and servings of different categories of foods recommended for people in risk category level 2 (mild risk).

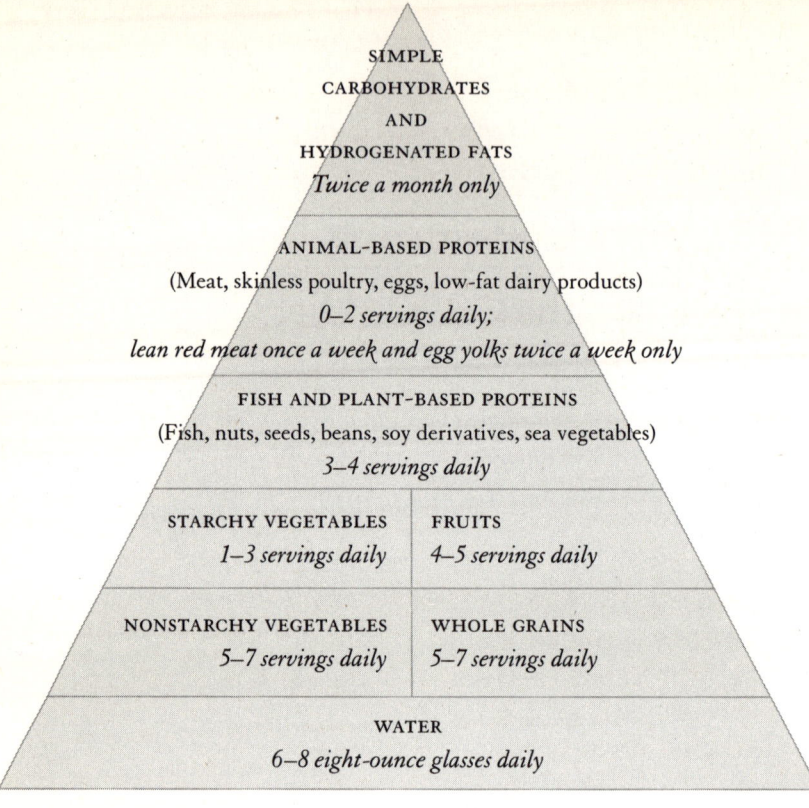

Figure 11.1 The Mild-Risk Food Pyramid

SPECIAL CONSIDERATIONS

- *Nonstarchy vegetables.* You can eat an unlimited amount of these vegetables, with a minimum of five to seven servings per day. I urge you to include a serving of sprouts, although this is not essential.
- *Whole grains.* Remember that whole grains introduce fiber into your system, and fiber facilitates the elimination of excess LDL cholesterol. So the higher your risk category, the more fiber you should be eating.
- *Fruits.* You need extra phytonutrients, so have between four and five servings of fruit each day.

- *Animal-based proteins.* You should have no more than two servings each day of an animal-based protein food. If you choose to eat dairy products, please make sure you always select low-fat varieties. If you eat poultry, make sure that it is skinless. You may eat one serving of lean red meat per week and egg yolks twice a week if you wish.

Level 3: Moderate Risk

Figure 11.2 illustrates the proportions and servings of different categories of foods recommended for people in risk category level 3 (moderate risk).

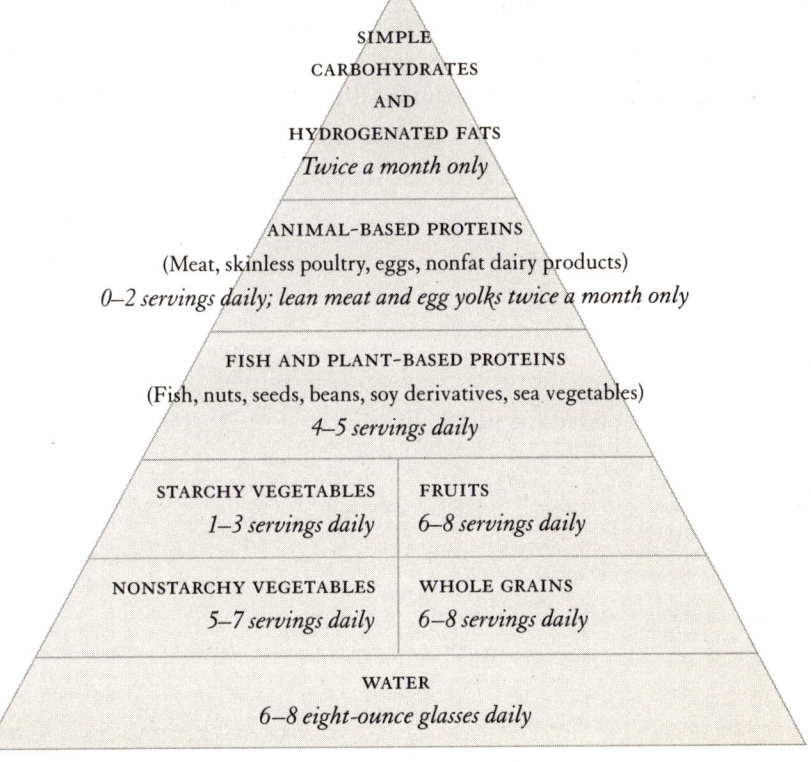

Figure 11.2 The Moderate-Risk Food Pyramid

SPECIAL CONSIDERATIONS

- *Nonstarchy vegetables.* If you are on the moderate-risk diet, you can eat an unlimited number of servings of nonstarchy vegetables. But you must be sure to include *at least* five to seven servings each day and at least one serving of sprouts.
- *Whole grains.* You need lots of extra complex carbohydrates, so I advise eating six to eight servings of whole grains and whole-grain products each day.
- *Animal-based proteins.* You need to be more careful about animal-based products than do people at lower risk levels. Yes, you may also have two servings daily of animal products, but you should use only nonfat items—skim milk, egg whites, and nonfat yogurt and cheeses. Also, please remember that some manufacturers try to give nonfat items a creamy texture by using chemical additives. Chemicals can increase the free radicals in your body and compound the unfortunate drama that is already taking place within your arteries. So be sure to read ingredients carefully and avoid nonfat products that aren't completely natural.

Level 4: High Risk

Figure 11.3 illustrates the proportions and servings of different categories of foods recommended for people in risk category level 4 (high risk).

Customizing the CARE Diet · 145

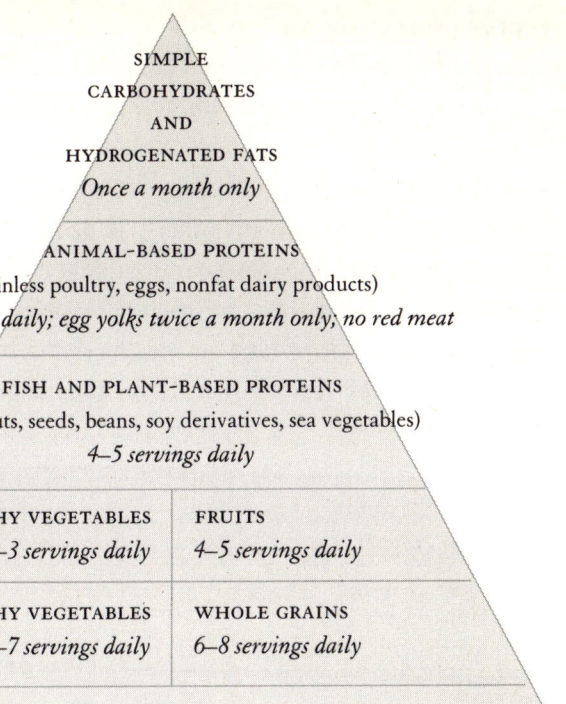

Figure 11.3 The High-Risk Food Pyramid

SPECIAL CONSIDERATIONS

- *Nonstarchy vegetables.* The more vegetables the merrier! You should have at least five to seven servings daily, but I advise you to make your servings closer to seven than to five. You should be sure to have one serving of sprouts each day as well.
- *Whole grains.* Like your moderate-risk counterparts, you should have at least six to eight servings of whole grains on a daily basis—and again, it's better to be closer to eight than to six.
- *Animal-based proteins.* Your recommended intake of animal-based protein is limited to one serving each day. In addition, you should avoid red meat completely and limit your consumption

of egg yolks to two per month. You can eat as many egg whites as you like, however. When it comes to dairy products, use only nonfat varieties and read labels carefully to make sure that the products you choose are free of chemical additives.

- *Simple carbohydrates and hydrogenated fats.* You have to be more careful than people in any other risk group. You can indulge in the items in this category no more than once a month. I suggest saving your treats for very special occasions. For example, you can have one slice of cake on your birthday, or a piece of turkey with sweetened cranberry sauce on Thanksgiving.

TIPS FOR PHYTO-FEASTING

Old habits are hard to break. Here are some tips to help you start making your diet richer in heart-healthy plant nutrients:

- Increase your serving sizes of vegetables.
- Snack on fresh fruit or vegetable "finger foods" (carrots, celery, pepper sticks, cherry tomatoes) instead of candy, pretzels, or chips.
- Include beans in your stews, soups, and pasta dishes.
- Sprinkle flaxseeds onto your cereals or salads and include them in meat loaves and casseroles.
- Flavor your foods with herbs and spices, such as ginger, rosemary, thyme, garlic, parsley, basil, and chives. This makes them more interesting, tasty, and nutritious.
- Add vegetables such as mushrooms, peppers, tomatoes, onions, and spinach as well as herbs when you are making an omelette.
- Drink water, tea, herbal tea, or 100 percent fruit or vegetable juices instead of soda.
- Add sautéed mushrooms, onions, garlic, and peppers to whole-grain dishes such as rice, barley, millet, couscous, or buckwheat.
- Put diced tofu in salads and add mashed tofu to casseroles.
- Add sea vegetables to scrambled eggs, stews, casseroles, and potpies.

- Wrap brown rice and vegetables in nori (a sea vegetable) to make delicious finger-food snacks.
- Buy an electric slow-cooker such as a Crock-Pot. Cut up and place the ingredients of your nutritious stew into the pot at night, then refrigerate. Turn on the pot before you leave for work and you will come home to a delicious, hearty dinner that's all ready for you.
- Vary your preparation of vegetables between raw, steamed, sautéed, boiled, blanched, and stir-fried. Make sure not to overcook your vegetables. This causes them to lose taste, texture, and nutritional content.
- Choose fresh vegetables as your first choice. Frozen is next best. Avoid any canned vegetables, which are the least desirable.

Special Needs

An additional factor in personalizing your diet involves taking into account specific health conditions that may affect you. Following are some notes for specific populations.

DIABETES

If you have diabetes, you need to work together with your health-care provider on further customizing the diet to your needs. As you know, people who have diabetes need to manage diet very carefully, especially the quantities of carbohydrates they eat and the timing of meals. You also need to modify your fruit intake and avoid dried fruits, since they are high in concentrated sugar. This type of management is best undertaken in close cooperation with a qualified health professional.

HIGH BLOOD PRESSURE

If you have high blood pressure, you need to reduce your sodium intake. This includes not only salt but also any food product that is high in sodium. Fortunately, sodium content is one of the items that must be listed on food product labels, so you can find out how much sodium a packaged food contains by reading the label. Please note that fresh, raw celery is extremely high in sodium, as is baking soda.

MENOPAUSE

If you are peri- or postmenopausal, you should include in your diet at least one serving of a soy product or chickpeas (garbanzo beans) every day to provide you with much-needed phytoestrogens. You should also emphasize foods that are rich in calcium.

ANEMIA

If you have been diagnosed with anemia, you should be emphasizing foods that are especially rich in iron, including spinach and other green leafy vegetables, fish, legumes, and whole grains. Iron is also present in sea vegetables, such as arame, dulse, hijiki, kombu, nori, and wakame. Depending on your level of risk—that is, whether you are allowed animal protein—you might chose lean red meat or eggs as sources of protein, since these contain large quantities of iron.

ORAL CONTRACEPTIVE USE

If you are taking birth control pills, you need extra sources of folic acid, because birth control pills are known to leach this substance from the body. Emphasize green leafy vegetables, legumes, whole wheat, and yeast. If you are allowed animal protein, you might want to include pork and lamb, which are high in folic acid.

OVERWEIGHT

If you are trying to lose weight, you need to be very conscious of your intake of nuts and carbohydrates—especially fruits, both fresh and dried.

Putting It All Together

Now it's time to organize your week. At the end of this chapter, you will find a series of sample menus that will help you get started. There is one set of suggested menus for each risk category. Remember that one food can fall into several nutritional categories and fulfill the requirement for all of them. For example, collard greens, which are highly nutritious, are (1) a vegetable; (2) a cruciferous vegetable; and (3) a dark leafy green vegetable. Chickpeas (garbanzo beans) are (1) a complex carbohydrate; (2) an excellent source of protein; and (3) a food rich in phytoestrogens, which are especially important for postmenopausal women.

Remember too that certain dishes can combine a large number of foods from several categories. Stew, for example, can have a base of meat, poultry, tofu, or seitan. It can also contain many different beans (such as kidney, lima, azuki), vegetables (onions, garlic, carrots, celery); whole grains (rice, barley); and sea vegetables (wakame, arame). Thus, a single easy-to-prepare dish can amount to one-stop shopping for many of your daily dietary requirements.

SERVING SIZES

You don't have to run around with a measuring cup, ruler, or scale, but it is important to get a sense of what correct serving sizes are. At least for the first couple of weeks, you should try to measure your foods. After that, it will become second nature and you can more easily guesstimate serving sizes.

In America, servings of some foods are getting larger and larger. The typical restaurant "serving" of French fries, for example, can be several times what a nutritionist would qualify as one serving. And many people *underestimate* what constitutes a serving of vegetables. One serving of vegetables does *not* mean one baby carrot, one stalk of celery, or one floret of broccoli. (When I ask my daughter to eat her vegetables, she looks at me innocently, brandishing a tiny tomato, and says, "But I'm eating *lots* of vegetables!") So it is necessary to have a realistic, if rough, sense of quantities.

Table 11.1 provides a list of many common foods and the amount that can be considered a single serving for each. Please note that the foods are classified according to their usual locations in the supermarket and how people commonly regard them. For example, botanically, a peanut is not actually a nut, but a legume; avocados and tomatoes are not vegetables, but fruits; mushrooms are not vegetables, but fungi. But because we think of peanuts as nuts and avocados, tomatoes, and mushrooms as vegetables, they are included in those categories here.

A note about cereals: You can obtain many high-fiber cereals from large name-brand companies, such as Kellogg's and General Mills. Unfortunately, these products usually are also extremely high in refined sugar, so I don't advise them. I suggest that you compare fiber *and* sugar contents. For a cereal to qualify as whole-grain, it should have at least 5 grams of fiber per serving, usually 1 cup.

Table 11.1
Serving Sizes for Selected Foods

Food Item	Single Serving Size
NONSTARCHY VEGETABLES	
Alfalfa sprouts	1 cup
Artichoke	1 small artichoke
Arugula	1 ounce
Asparagus	5 spears
Bok choy (Chinese cabbage)	½ cup shredded
Broccoli:	
fresh	1 medium spear raw; 1 cup cooked
frozen	½ cup cooked
Brussels sprouts	1 cup raw (about 3 sprouts); ½ cup cooked
Cabbage	1 cup raw, ½ cup cooked
Carrots:	
baby	10 carrots
regular	1 medium carrot raw; 1 cup cooked
Cauliflower	3 medium florets raw; 1 cup cooked
Celery	2 medium stalks
Chicory greens	½ cup chopped
Chicory root	1 medium root
Collard greens	½ cup chopped
Cucumber	½ cup sliced
Daikon (Chinese radish)	½ cup sliced
Dandelion greens	½ cup raw, chopped
Eggplant	½ cup cubed, cooked; 4 slices (about 7 ounces) sliced, cooked
Endive	1 cup raw
Green beans	½ cup

(continued)

Food Item	Single Serving Size
NONSTARCHY VEGETABLES	
Green salad	2 cups (⅗ ounce)
Kale	½ cup raw, chopped
Kohlrabi	½ cup raw, sliced
Leeks	1 medium leek (about 4½ ounces) cooked
Lettuce	1 cup shredded
Mushrooms	4 ounces
Mustard greens	1 cup
Okra	½ cup (about 8 pods)
Onion	1 small onion
Parsley	1 cup raw, chopped
Peppers (green, red, or yellow)	1 medium raw; 1 cup raw, chopped
Radish	10 medium raw; ½ cup cooked
Rhubarb	½ cup
Rutabaga	½ cup raw, cubed, or cooked, mashed
Spinach	3 ounces (about 1½ cups) raw; 1 cup cooked
Squash, summer	½ cup (about 4¼ ounces)
Swiss chard	½ cup
Tomato:	
cherry	5 tomatoes
regular	1 medium raw; ½ cup cooked
Watercress	½ cup cooked or raw
WHOLE GRAINS AND GRAIN PRODUCTS	
Amaranth	1 cup uncooked
Barley	1 cup cooked
Bread, whole-grain	1 slice
Bread crumbs	½ cup
Bulgur	½ cup cooked

Food Item	Single Serving Size
WHOLE GRAINS AND GRAIN PRODUCTS	
Cereal, whole-grain:	
Bran flakes	⅔ cup dry
Fiber One	1 cup dry
Kamut flakes	1 cup dry
Multigrain flakes	1 cup dry
Oat bran	⅓–½ cup dry
Oatmeal	1 cup cooked
Puffed corn	1 cup dry
Wheat bran	1 cup dry
Wheatena	½ cup cooked
Couscous	1 cup cooked
Kasha (buckwheat groats)	⅓ cup cooked
Millet	½ cup cooked
Pasta, whole-grain	1 cup (2 ounces) cooked
Pretzels, whole-wheat	2 medium pretzels; 10 twists (2 ounces)
Quinoa	½ cup cooked
Rice, brown	½ cup cooked
Spelt	1 ounce cooked
Teff	¼ cup (about 1½ ounces) cooked
Wild rice	1 cup cooked
FRUIT AND FRUIT JUICES	
Apple	1 small apple
Apricots	3 medium apricots, fresh; ½ cup dried
Banana	1 medium banana
Blackberries	1 cup
Black currants	1 cup
Blueberries	1 cup
Cantaloupe	¼ medium melon *(continued)*

Food Item	Single Serving Size
FRUIT AND FRUIT JUICES	
Cherries	10 medium cherries
Clementines	2 medium clementines
Cranberries	1 cup fresh, chopped; ½ cup dried
Dates	¼ cup dried, chopped
Elderberries	1 cup
Figs	1 medium fig, fresh; ½ cup dried
Gooseberries	1 cup
Grapefruit	1 small grapefruit
Grapefruit juice	1 cup
Grapes	1½ cups
Grape juice	1 cup
Guava	1 cup
Honeydew	¹⁄₁₀ medium melon, sliced; 1 cup cubed
Kiwi	2 medium kiwis
Kumquats	1 medium kumquat
Mango	1 medium mango
Nectarines	1 medium nectarine
Olives	4 medium olives; 3 extra-large olives
Orange	1 medium orange
Orange juice (freshly squeezed)	1 cup
Papaya	½ medium papaya; 1 cup cubed
Peach	2 small peaches
Pear	1 medium pear
Pineapple	2 medium slices; ½ cup chunks
Plum	2 small plums
Prunes	1 cup dried
Raisins	¼ cup
Raspberries	1 cup
Strawberries	1 cup

Food Item	Single Serving Size
FRUIT AND FRUIT JUICES	
Tangerines	1 medium tangerine
Watermelon	1 inch x 10-inch diameter slice
STARCHY VEGETABLES	
Avocado	1 medium avocado; 1 cup mashed
Beets	½ cup cooked
Corn:	
kernels	½ cup cooked
on the cob	1 medium ear
Parsnip	⅔ cup cooked
Popcorn (air-popped)	3 cups
Potato	1 medium potato, baked; ½ cup mashed
Squash, winter	½ cup cooked
Sweet potato	1 medium sweet potato
Turnips	½ cup cooked, mashed, or cubed
Yams	½ cup cooked
FISH AND SEA PROTEIN	
Bass	3 ounces cooked
Crab	1 leg or 3–5 ounces, cooked
Crayfish	3 ounces or 8 fish, raw
Eel	½ fillet (3 ounces) cooked
Flounder	1 fillet (4½ ounces) fresh, cooked
Haddock	1 fillet (about 5⅓ ounces) fresh, cooked
Halibut	½ fillet (about 5½ ounces) fresh, cooked
Lobster	1 medium lobster, cooked
Mackerel	1 fillet (about 5 ounces) cooked
Oysters	6 medium; ½ cup

(continued)

Food Item	Single Serving Size
FISH AND SEA PROTEIN	
Pike	½ fillet (about 5½ ounces) fresh, cooked
Roe	3 ounces cooked
Salmon:	
canned	3 ounces
fresh	½ fillet (about 5½ ounces) cooked
Sardines, canned	1 can (3.3 ounces)
Sea vegetables:	
Agar	1 ounce
Arame	½ cup (about ⅓ ounce)
Dulse	⅓ cup (7 grams) dried; 1 ounce flakes
Hijiki	½ cup (about ⅓ ounce)
Kelp	1 ounce
Kombu	1 ounce
Nori	1 ounce
Wakame	1 ounce
Shrimp	4 large shrimp, cooked
Snapper	½ fillet (3 ounces) cooked
Sole	1 fillet (4½ ounces) cooked
Tilefish	½ fillet (about 5⅓ ounces) cooked
Trout	3 ounces cooked
Tuna, canned	½ can (3 ounces)
BEANS, LEGUMES, AND LEGUME PRODUCTS	
Beans (aduki, black, kidney, lima, soy, etc.)	⅓ – ½ cup cooked
Black-eyed peas	⅓ cup cooked
Chickpeas (garbanzo beans)	½ cup cooked
Falafel	3 balls
Hummus (chickpea paste)	½ cup
Lentils	½ cup cooked

Food Item	Single Serving Size
BEANS, LEGUMES, AND LEGUME PRODUCTS	
Peas, green	½ – ⅔ cup fresh
Soybeans and soy products:	
miso	1 tablespoon
miso soup	1 cup
soybeans	½ cup cooked; 1 ounce roasted and toasted
soy butter, roasted	2 tablespoons
soy cheese	
American type	1 slice (¾ ounce)
cream cheese	2 tablespoons
other types	1 ounce
soy flour	¼ cup
soy hot dog	2 hot dogs
soymilk	6–8 ounces
soy nuts	¼ cup
tempeh	½ cup
textured vegetable protein (TVP):	
beef style, chunks or ground	3 ½ ounces
dry	¼ cup
tofu	3–4 ounces
tofu yogurt	1 cup
Veggie burger	1 patty (2–3½ ounces)
NUTS AND NUT PRODUCTS	
Almonds	1 ounce
Brazil nuts	1 ounce
Cashews	1 ounce
Chestnuts	1 ounce (2–3 nuts)
Hazelnuts (filberts)	1 ounce

(continued)

Food Item	Single Serving Size
NUTS AND NUT PRODUCTS	
Macadamia nuts	1 ounce
Nut butters	2 tablespoons
Peanuts, dry-roasted	1 ounce
Pecans	1 ounce
Pine nuts	1 ounce
Pistachios	1 ounce
Walnuts	1 ounce
SEEDS AND SEED PRODUCTS	
Flaxseeds	2 tablespoons ground
Pumpkinseeds	1 ounce
Sesame seeds	1 tablespoon
Sunflower seeds	1 ounce
Tahini (sesame seed paste)	1 tablespoon
MEAT, POULTRY, AND MEAT AND POULTRY PRODUCTS	
Bacon	3 strips cooked
Beef	3 ounces cooked
Beef jerky	1 piece (about ⅔ ounce)
Beerwurst	1 slice (1 ounce)
Bologna	1 slice (1 ounce)
Chicken	½ medium breast or back, 2 small drumsticks, or 1 whole leg, cooked
Duck	6 ounces skinless, cooked
Elk	3 ounces cooked
Ham	3 ounces extra lean, boneless, roasted; 3 slices (about 2¼ ounces) baked

Food Item	Single Serving Size
MEAT, POULTRY, AND MEAT AND POULTRY PRODUCTS	
Hot dog	1 hot dog
Lamb	3 ounces or 2 chops cooked
Pastrami	2 ounces
Pheasant	½ breast or 2 legs cooked, or 1 leg or ¼ breast cooked
Pork	3 ounces cooked
Rabbit	3 ounces cooked
Salami	2 ounces
Turkey:	
dark meat	3 ounces skinless, roasted
light meat	4 ounces skinless, roasted
Venison	3 ounces roasted
DAIRY PRODUCTS AND EGGS	
American cheese	1 slice (1 ounce)
Blue cheese	1 ounce
Brie	1 ounce
Butter	1 tablespoon
Camembert	1⅓ ounces
Cheddar cheese	1 ounce
Colby cheese	1 ounce
Cottage cheese	½ cup
Cream cheese	2 tablespoons (about 1 ounce)
Eggs	1 egg
Feta cheese	1 ounce
Gouda	1 ounce
Gruyère	1 ounce
Milk	1 cup
Monterey Jack cheese	1 ounce

(continued)

Food Item	Single Serving Size
DAIRY PRODUCTS AND EGGS	
Mozzarella	1 ounce
Muenster cheese	1 ounce
Parmesan cheese	1 ounce
Provolone	1 ounce
Ricotta cheese:	
part skim	1 cup
whole milk	½ cup
Romano cheese	1 ounce
Roquefort	1 ounce
Swiss cheese	1 ounce
Yogurt	8 ounces
REFINED FLOUR PRODUCTS	
Bagel	1 bagel
Cake	1 slice
Cereal, non-whole-grain:	
Cheerios	1 cup dry
Corn flakes	1¼ cups (1 ounce) dry
Farina	¾ cup cooked
Special K	1 cup dry
Muffin	1 muffin
Pasta	1 cup cooked
White bread	2 slices
White rice	¾ cup cooked

Food Item	Single Serving Size
SPREADS, CONDIMENTS, AND MISCELLANEOUS	
Ginger	¼ fresh root; 1 teaspoon ground
Margarine	1 tablespoon
Mayonnaise	1 tablespoon
Salad dressing	1–2 tablespoons
Seitan	3½ ounces

SAMPLE MENUS

Creating a new dietary lifestyle can be very challenging. What can I eat? What should I cook? Following are daily menus that are designed to help you get started. Remember that these are merely samples and recommendations. You can substitute items that better suit your taste, lifestyle, and the season of the year based on the guidelines in this chapter.

Note that, unless otherwise specified, each item in the menus refers to a single serving.

Sample Daily Menus for Level 1, Prevention

	Monday	Tuesday	Wednesday	Thursday	Friday	Saturday	Sunday
BREAKFAST	Wheatena cooked with milk Sliced banana Tea with lemon	Freshly squeezed orange juice Omelette made with 2 eggs, peppers, tomatoes, mushrooms, onions, and wakame 2 slices whole-wheat toast Tea with soymilk	Whole oatmeal, cooked with soymilk Raisins and dried cranberries Sliced peach	Cottage cheese sprinkled with flaxseeds and almonds Sliced pear Oat bran muffin Green tea	Bran flakes with milk, sprinkled with pecans and sliced banana	French toast made with 2 slices whole-wheat bread, egg whites, and milk or soymilk Grapefruit juice Sliced strawberries	Pancakes made with whole-wheat flour, eggs, and milk or soymilk Unsweetened fruit preserves Nectarine Green tea
MIDMORNING SNACK	Baby carrots	Soy nuts Herbal tea	Whole-wheat crackers with almond butter	Pumpkin seeds Whole-grain pretzels Herbal tea	Homemade trail mix made with soy nuts, almonds, sunflower seeds, and raisins	Baked corn chips dipped in cashew butter	Air-popped popcorn Soy chips Tomato juice
LUNCH	Sandwich made with 2 slices whole-wheat bread; tuna salad made with soy mayonnaise,	Salad made with chickpeas, sprouts, and buckwheat	Veggie burger with ketchup, lettuce, and a pickle on a whole-grain roll	Salmon Millet and brown rice Arugula and endives	Whole-grain bread with hummus Lettuce and tomato Couscous	Bulgur wheat salad with sprouts Soy veggie burger with ketchup	Tofu pizza with tomatoes, peppers, onions, and mushrooms

chopped celery, and chopped onion or scallion; lettuce; and sliced tomato Low-sugar, low-fat coleslaw Plum	Cantaloupe	Zucchini	Tabbouleh			Carrot juice

AFTERNOON SNACK

Sliced peppers Tomato juice	Carrot and celery sticks Grapes	Baby carrots	Sliced peppers	Cherry tomatoes	Soy chips Apple	Blueberries

DINNER

Beef stew made with kidney beans, potato, onion, celery, carrot, garlic, and hijiki Brown rice Salad sprinkled with sunflower seeds and flaxseeds	Tofu sautéed with mushrooms, onion, garlic, and whole-wheat pasta Steamed broccoli Corn on the cob	Seitan stew made with onion, garlic, potato, carrot, and sea vegetables Peas and beans	Miso soup with whole-wheat noodles and arame Sweet potato Chicken Kale	Halibut Mashed potatoes Collard greens Asparagus	Salmon Sweet potato Salad sprinkled with flaxseeds and walnuts Spinach	Lentil soup made with potato, sea vegetables, carrots, celery, mushrooms, onions, and garlic Stir-fry with tofu, snow peas, green peppers, and onions Brown rice

DESSERT OR EVENING SNACK

Sliced orange	Soy yogurt with mixed berries	Strawberries	Sorbet (pure fruit) with kiwi	Grapefruit	Watermelon	Sliced pineapple

Sample Daily Menus for Level 2, Low Risk

	MONDAY	TUESDAY	WEDNESDAY	THURSDAY	FRIDAY	SATURDAY	SUNDAY
BREAKFAST	Wheatena cooked with low-fat milk Sliced banana Tea with lemon	Freshly squeezed orange juice Omelette made with 2 eggs, peppers, tomatoes, mushrooms, onions, and wakame 2 slices whole-wheat toast Tea with soymilk	Whole oatmeal cooked with soymilk Raisins and dried cranberries Sliced peach	Low-fat cottage cheese sprinkled with flaxseeds and almonds Sliced pear Oat bran muffin Green tea	Bran flakes with low-fat milk, sprinkled with pecans and sliced banana	French toast made with 2 slices whole-wheat bread, egg whites, and low-fat milk or soymilk Grapefruit juice Sliced strawberries	Pancakes made with whole-wheat flour, eggs, and low-fat milk or soymilk Unsweetened fruit preserves Nectarine Green tea
MIDMORNING SNACK	Baby carrots Pear	Soy nuts Herbal tea Clementine	Whole-wheat crackers with almond butter	Pumpkin seeds Whole-grain pretzels Herbal tea	Homemade trail mix made with soy nuts, almonds, sunflower seeds, and raisins	Baked corn chips dipped in cashew butter Blueberries	Air-popped popcorn Soy chips Tomato juice
LUNCH	Sandwich made with 2 slices whole-wheat bread; tuna salad made with soy mayonnaise, chopped celery, and chopped onion or scallion;	Salad made with chickpeas, sprouts, and buckwheat	Veggie burger with ketchup, lettuce, and a pickle on a whole-grain roll Cantaloupe	Salmon Millet and brown rice Arugula and endives Zucchini	Whole-grain bread with hummus Lettuce and tomato Couscous Tabbouleh	Bulgur wheat salad with sprouts Soy veggie burger with ketchup	Tofu pizza with tomatoes, peppers, onions, and mushrooms Carrot juice

lettuce; and sliced tomato Low-sugar, low-fat coleslaw Plum						

AFTERNOON SNACK

Sliced peppers Tomato juice	Carrot and celery sticks Grapes	Baby carrots	Sliced peppers	Cherry tomatoes	Soy chips Apple	Blueberries Raspberries

DINNER

Beef stew made with kidney beans, potato, onion, celery, carrot, garlic, and hijiki Brown rice Salad sprinkled with sunflower seeds and flaxseeds	Tofu sautéed with mushrooms, onion, garlic, and whole-wheat pasta Steamed broccoli Corn on the cob	Seitan stew made with onion, garlic, potato, carrot, and sea vegetables Peas and beans Bok choy	Miso soup with whole-wheat noodles and arame Sweet potato Lean chicken Kale	Halibut Mashed potatoes Collard greens Asparagus	Salmon Sweet potato Salad sprinkled with flaxseeds and walnuts Spinach	Lentil soup with potatoes, sea vegetables, carrots, celery, mushrooms, onions, and garlic Stir-fry with tofu, snow peas, green peppers, and onions Brown rice

DESSERT OR EVENING SNACK

Sliced orange	Soy yogurt with mixed berries	Strawberries	Sorbet (pure fruit) with kiwi Honeydew	Grapefruit	Watermelon Whole-wheat crackers	Sliced pineapple

Sample Daily Menus for Level 3, Moderate Risk

	Monday	Tuesday	Wednesday	Thursday	Friday	Saturday	Sunday
Breakfast	Wheatena cooked with nonfat milk and oat bran; Sliced banana; Tea with lemon	Freshly squeezed orange juice; Omelette made with 2 egg whites, peppers, tomatoes, mushrooms, onions, and wakame; 2 slices whole-wheat toast; Tea with soymilk	Whole oatmeal cooked with soymilk and oat bran; Raisins and dried cranberries; Sliced peach	Nonfat cottage cheese sprinkled with flaxseeds and almonds; Sliced pear; Oat bran muffin; Green tea	Bran flakes with nonfat milk, sprinkled with pecans and sliced banana	French toast made with 2 slices whole-wheat bread, egg whites, and nonfat milk, or soymilk; Grapefruit juice; Sliced strawberries	Pancakes made with whole-wheat flour, egg whites, and nonfat milk or soymilk; Unsweetened fruit preserves; Nectarine; Green tea
Midmorning Snack	Baby carrots; Pear	Soy nuts; Herbal tea; Clementine	Whole-wheat crackers with almond butter	Pumpkin seeds; Whole-grain pretzels; Herbal tea	Homemade trail mix made with soy nuts, almonds, sunflower seeds, low-fat rolled-oat granola, and raisins	Baked corn chips and whole-wheat crackers dipped in cashew butter; Blueberries	Air-popped popcorn; Soy chips; Tomato juice
Lunch	Sandwich made with 2 slices whole-wheat bread; tuna salad made with soy mayonnaise, chopped	Salad made with chickpeas, sprouts, and buckwheat sprinkled with rice bran	Veggie burger with ketchup, lettuce, and pickle on a whole-grain roll; Cantaloupe	Salmon; Millet and brown rice; Arugula and endive	Whole-grain bread with hummus; Lettuce and tomato; Couscous	Bulgur wheat salad with sprouts; Soy veggie burger with ketchup	Tofu pizza with tomatoes, peppers, onions, and mushrooms; Carrot juice

celery, and chopped onion or scallion; lettuce; and sliced tomato Low-sugar, low-fat coleslaw Plum			Zucchini Tabbouleh			Baked zucchini breaded with whole-wheat crumbs

AFTERNOON SNACK

Sliced peppers Tomato juice	Carrot and celery sticks Grapes	Baby carrots	Sliced peppers	Cherry tomatoes	Soy chips Apple	Blueberries Raspberries

DINNER

Stew made with aduki beans, kidney beans, potato, onion, celery, carrot, garlic, and hijiki Brown rice Lean turkey slices Salad sprinkled with sunflower seeds and flaxseeds	Tofu sautéed with mushrooms, onion, garlic, and whole-wheat pasta Steamed broccoli Corn on the cob	Seitan stew made with onion, garlic, potato, carrot, and sea vegetables Peas and beans Bok choy	Miso soup with whole-wheat noodles and arame Sweet potato Lean chicken Kale	Halibut Mashed potatoes Kasha (buckwheat groats) Collard greens Asparagus	Salmon Sweet potato Salad sprinkled with flaxseeds and walnuts Spinach	Lentil soup with potatoes, sea vegetables, carrots, celery, mushrooms, onions, and garlic Stir-fry with tofu, snow peas, green peppers, and onions Brown rice

DESSERT OR EVENING SNACK

Sliced orange	Soy yogurt with mixed berries	Strawberries	Sorbet (pure fruit) with kiwi Honeydew	Grapefruit	Watermelon Whole-wheat crackers	Sliced pineapple

Sample Daily Menus for Level 4, High Risk

	Monday	Tuesday	Wednesday	Thursday	Friday	Saturday	Sunday
BREAKFAST	Wheatena cooked with soymilk and oat bran Sliced banana Tea with lemon	Freshly squeezed orange juice Omelette made with 2 egg whites, peppers, tomatoes, mushrooms, onions, and wakame 2 slices whole-wheat toast Tea with soymilk	Whole oatmeal cooked with soymilk, oat bran, raisins, and dried cranberries Sliced peach	Nonfat cottage cheese sprinkled with flaxseeds and almonds Sliced pear Oat bran muffin Green tea	Bran flakes with soymilk sprinkled with pecans and sliced banana	French toast made with 2 slices whole-wheat bread, egg whites, and nonfat milk or soymilk Grapefruit juice Sliced strawberries	Pancakes made with whole-wheat flour, egg whites, and nonfat milk or soymilk Unsweetened fruit preserves Nectarine Green tea
MIDMORNING SNACK	Baby carrots Pear	Soy nuts Herbal tea Clementine	Whole-wheat crackers with almond butter	Pumpkin seeds Whole-grain pretzels Herbal tea	Homemade trail mix made with soy nuts, almonds, sunflower seeds, low-fat rolled-oat granola, and raisins	Baked corn chips and whole-wheat crackers dipped in cashew butter Blueberries	Air-popped popcorn Soy chips Tomato juice
LUNCH	Sandwich made with 2 slices whole-wheat bread; tuna salad made with soy mayonnaise, chopped celery,	Salad made with chickpeas, sprouts, and buckwheat, sprinkled with rice bran	Veggie burger with ketchup, lettuce, and pickle on a whole-grain roll Cantaloupe	Salmon Millet and brown rice Arugula and endive	Whole-grain bread with hummus Lettuce and tomato Couscous	Bulgur wheat salad with sprouts Soy veggie burger with ketchup	Tofu pizza with tomatoes, peppers, onions, and mushrooms

and chopped onion or scallion; lettuce; and sliced tomato								Zucchini	Carrot juice
Low-sugar, low-fat coleslaw								Tabbouleh	Baked zucchini breaded with whole-wheat crumbs
Plum									

AFTERNOON SNACK

Sliced peppers	Carrot and celery sticks	Baby carrots	Sliced peppers	Cherry tomatoes	Soy chips	Blueberries
Tomato juice	Grapes				Apple	Raspberries

DINNER

Stew made with aduki beans, kidney beans, potato, onion, celery, carrot, garlic, and hijiki	Tofu sautéed with mushrooms, onion, garlic, and whole-wheat pasta	Seitan stew made with onion, garlic, potato, carrot, and sea vegetables	Miso soup with whole-wheat noodles and arame	Halibut	Salmon	Lentil soup with potatoes, sea vegetables, carrots, celery, mushrooms, onions, and garlic
Brown rice	Steamed broccoli	Peas and beans	Sweet potato	Mashed potatoes	Sweet potato	Stir-fry with tofu, snow peas, green peppers, and onion
Lean turkey slices	Corn on the cob	Bok choy	Textured vegetable protein with onions and garlic	Kasha (buckwheat groats)	Salad sprinkled with flaxseeds and walnuts	Brown rice
Salad sprinkled with sunflower seeds and flaxseeds			Kale	Collard greens	Spinach	
				Asparagus		

DESSERT OR EVENING SNACK

Sliced orange	Soy yogurt with mixed berries	Strawberries	Sorbet (pure fruit) with kiwi	Grapefruit	Watermelon	Sliced pineapple
			Honeydew		Whole-wheat crackers	

Some Final Tips

Most of us have established ways of eating. Changing your diet and keeping track of what you eat is challenging. In chapter 15, we will discuss what you can do to overcome some common obstacles, and chapter 16 will provide you with the basis for creating a personal workbook to help you keep track of your diet and other components of your new lifestyle.

Finally, if you slip and allow yourself foods that are not in accordance with these guidelines, don't despair. It's never too late to change, and sometimes change can take place only gradually. Keep trying.

12 Supplements That Care for Your Heart

There is more to life than food.
—Anonymous

Even if your diet were ideal, you would still need some form of nutritional supplementation to ensure an adequate supply of all necessary nutrients. This is so because a variety of circumstances converge to compromise the nutritional value of our produce and whole grains. These include growing conditions, shipping conditions, the method of storage and length of time the food is stored, and the rapid-ripening procedures to which some of our produce is subjected. Certainly, supplements are absolutely essential for individuals with a systemic imbalance or disorders, such as elevated cholesterol, homocysteine, or CRP levels, as well as for people who engage in regular strenuous exercise, people who are exposed to environmental toxins or pesticides, people who smoke or are exposed to secondhand smoke, people who have illnesses or infections or who are recovering from significant physical or emotional traumas, pregnant women and nursing mothers, and people who take certain medications—especially many of the medications used for cardiovascular conditions. This chapter will focus on the supplements you need to address your cardiovascular health.

We will begin with supplements that support all people's health, whether or not they have heart or circulatory problems. These supplements work preventively and are good for general health maintenance. Then we will look at supplements that specifically address elevated cholesterol levels. These agents can be used as alternatives to statin drugs. Finally, we will cover supplements that promote cardiovascular health through mechanisms other than cholesterol reduction.

As with the CARE diet, it is useful to organize supplement programs around levels of risk. If you have a higher level of risk, you may need not only to take more types of supplements, but you may need to take higher dosages of the basic supplements, such as vitamin E or folic acid, than you would take if you were in a lower risk group.

You will notice, too, that I never suggest a specific dose, but a range of dosages. Let me explain why:

- Even conventional medicines, such as cold and pain medications, do not give exact instructions. For example, you may be told to take two tablets every two to four hours, not to exceed six doses in a day.
- The ranges offer guidelines regarding the lowest dosage that is effective and the highest dosage that is safe to take without medical supervision. It is always wise to begin with the smallest dose and work upward. It is possible that you will obtain excellent results from small doses and that you won't need to use the maximum dose.
- Individual needs will differ depending on a person's age, weight, general medical condition, severity of symptoms, and other factors. No book can provide minute guidance for every possible contingency. (That's why it is best if you can work closely with a health-care provider who is well-versed in the use of nutritional supplements.)

- People tend to think that the dosing of conventional medications is a completely scientific, hard-and-fast process. This isn't the case. Most physicians will tell you that medication management is as much an art as a science, and a trial-and-error process is often required before arriving at the correct dosage, medication, or combination of medications. The same is true for natural supplementation.

Now let us move on to the specific recommendations. I think that everyone should take a basic vitamin/mineral supplement to make sure that all the minimum daily requirements of these important micronutrients are represented. If your risk is negligible (level 1), this is all you need on a regular basis. Table 12.1 shows what you should be looking for in a multivitamin and mineral supplement.

Follow the dosage instructions on the product label; these may vary depending on what brand you select. Please note that many manufacturers require you to take more than one tablet or capsule per day in order to obtain the nutritional value of the entire list of ingredients on the label.

TABLE 12.1
Recommended Nutrient Content of a Multivitamin and Mineral Supplement

Nutrient	Amount per Tablet
VITAMINS	
Vitamin A (including beta-carotene)	5,000–15,000 IU
Vitamin B_1 (thiamin)	50–100 mg
Vitamin B_2 (riboflavin)	50–100 mg
Vitamin B_3 (niacin/niacinamide)	50–100 mg
Vitamin B_6 (pyridoxine)	50–100 mg
Vitamin B_{12} (cobalamin)	50–100 mcg

(continued)

Folic acid	400–800 mcg
Biotin	10–75 mcg
Inositol	10–25 mg
Pantothenic acid	10–75 mg
Para-aminobenzoic acid (PABA)	10–70 mg
Vitamin C	500–1,000 mg
Vitamin D	400–800 IU
Vitamin E	150–600 IU
MINERALS	
Boron	0.5–3 mg
Calcium	250–500 mg
Chromium	25–200 mcg
Copper	0.5–2 mg
Iodine	50–150 mcg
Magnesium	100–250 mg
Manganese	1–15 mg
Selenium	25–200 mcg
Zinc	10–20 mg

Level 2: Mild-Risk Program

If you are in the mild-risk category, the following summarizes the supplements appropriate for you.

- *Multivitamin and mineral supplement* (see table 12.1). As with everyone, you should take a basic multivitamin and mineral supplement daily.
- *Vitamin C.* Take 1,000–2,000 mg daily. This is probably one of the most popular vitamin supplements. Vitamin C is a key antioxidant. It helps to raise levels of HDL cholesterol and lower

LDL levels by assaulting free radicals. It has been associated with a reduction in high blood pressure, and it also assists in the process of tissue repair and regrowth. Some studies have linked vitamin C with a reduction in homocysteine levels and the prevention of the LDL oxidization process, especially when taken in conjunction with the B vitamins and vitamin E. The regular use of vitamin C supplements can greatly reduce the risk of death from coronary artery disease. In one study, researchers administered 1,000 milligrams of vitamin C each day to their subjects. The incidence of death from coronary artery disease was reduced by 42 percent for men and 25 percent for women— extraordinarily impressive findings indeed!

Vitamin C is useful not only for cholesterol and homocysteine reduction but also for the prevention of restenosis after angioplasty. Studies have shown that taking even a modest dose (500 milligrams) of vitamin C can significantly reduce the risk of this problem.

Note: In rare instances, vitamin C can have a negative impact on the stomach, contributing to heartburn. If you have a history of hiatal hernia, ulcers, gastroesophageal reflux disease (GERD), heartburn, or other stomach disorders, consult your physician before using vitamin C supplements and be sure to use only *buffered* vitamin C, which has been mixed with minerals to protect the stomach lining from some of the erosive effects of the acid. It helps to take vitamin C on a full stomach. Also, some people experience intestinal gas and loose stools from very high doses of vitamin C. Again, taking the buffered form and being sure to take it with food should reduce these symptoms. Finally, although vitamin C is available in chewable form, it is advisable to use this only as an occasional treat rather than as your steady source of this important vitamin. The combined sugar and acid contents in the chewable tablet can leach calcium from your tooth enamel. The same is true of ascorbic acid powder. You can rinse your mouth briefly with baking soda just after taking these forms of vitamin C to help mitigate this effect.

- *Vitamin E.* Take 400–800 IU of mixed tocopherols and 50–200 mg of tocotrienols daily.

  There is hardly a nutrient on the market that has received as much publicity in recent years as vitamin E. In fact, it has been estimated that if everyone took adequate quantities of vitamin E, we could probably cut our health care costs by up to $8 billion per year. That's not bad for a substance that may cost less than 20 cents per day.

  Vitamin E is one of the greatest gifts you can give your cardiovascular system. In conjunction with vitamin C, it inhibits LDL oxidation and excessive blood clotting, and together with the B vitamin group it helps reduce homocysteine levels.

  Although we generally refer to vitamin E as if it were one substance, it actually consists of eight different *isomers,* or structural forms. *Vitamin E* is actually a generic term for this entire family of compounds. The two major compound groups within this family are called *tocopherols* and *tocotrienols.*

  In the tocopherol group, the most common are alpha-, beta-, delta-, and gamma-tocopherols, although alpha-tocopherol has received by far the most scientific attention. Perhaps there is good reason for this, because it appears that alpha-tocopherol has the highest antioxidant potential. Lately, gamma-tocopherol has begun to receive recognition as a potent antioxidant, too, which is why I am in favor of using supplements that contain all of the tocopherols.

  Some recent studies have called into question the value of high-dose vitamin E supplements in the reduction of CVD. However, many other studies contradict these findings. How do you know which studies are most accurate? My clinical experience bears out the benefits of vitamin E and confirms its use in the prevention and treatment of CVD. But vitamin E isn't just good for your heart and circulation. It's great for your immune system—especially for people over age sixty—and also for your skin. Interestingly, it helps in tissue maintenance and repair, so it is useful for people who are recovering from surgery or injuries. Finally, it helps to address symptoms of premenstrual syndrome (PMS). All in all, it is one of the most important and versatile vitamins in the arsenal.

Scientists have recently turned their attention to the tocotrienols—especially alpha-tocotrienol—as well, and are finding that they have significant antioxidant and other health benefits. Recently, tocotrienol-rich vitamin E supplements have become available.

Although tocotrienols have key antioxidant effects that are important for cancer prevention as well as the prevention of CVD, the most important benefit appears to be as a blood thinner. In a study of stroke survivors with atherosclerosis in their carotid arteries (the arteries that serve the brain), one-quarter of those who were given supplements rich in tocopherols and tocotrienols showed some reversal of their disease. Carotid plaque regressed, the degree of arterial narrowing and blockage decreased, and blood flow increased.

I generally recommend that my patients use both forms of vitamin E. When looking for tocopherol supplements, look for a product that contains *mixed tocopherols* rather than only the alpha variety. If you can find only supplements with alpha-tocopherol, at least try to opt for the more natural variety, which is d-alpha tocopheryl succinate, rather than dl-tocopheryl-acetate, which is a synthetic version. The succinate form of vitamin E is probably the best absorbed and utilized.

Who should take vitamin E? If you have any cardiovascular risk factors, especially high cholesterol or triglycerides, or high blood pressure, vitamin E will be helpful for you. Tocotrienols are especially helpful if you are recovering from a stroke. It can also help prevent inflammation.

Note: Because vitamin E has powerful blood-thinning and

antihypertensive effects, you should consult a health-care professional if you are taking anticoagulant or antihypertensive medications, or if you suffer from low blood pressure. People have safely used vitamin E along with those other medications, so long as they are taken at least six hours apart, but it is a good idea to ask your physician, who knows your own particular health profile. It is also a good idea to start with a low dosage (200 IU) and work up gradually to the desired level, rather than beginning abruptly with higher dosages. Also, extremely high dosages of vitamin E (over 1,600 IU daily) can cause nausea, diarrhea, flatulence, and even, in rare instances, fainting or heart palpitations. This is extremely unusual and totally reversible when the dosage is decreased. Finally, if you are planning to have surgery, you should stop taking vitamin E a week prior to the surgery, due to its blood-thinning effects.

- *Vitamin B-complex with folic acid* (see table 12.2). Each of the B vitamins performs a somewhat different function individually, and the entire group has been shown to work together synergistically. Additionally, B vitamins reduce the risk of heart attack and death from cardiac causes.

    Table 12.2 gives the nutritional content of an ideal B-complex supplement. You do not need to supplement with individual vitamins from the B group unless you are in the higher risk categories or have other specific medical needs.

Table 12.2
Recommended Nutrient Content of a B-Complex Supplement

Nutrient	Recommended Daily Dosage
Vitamin B_1 (thiamin)	50–100 mg
Vitamin B_2 (riboflavin)	50–100 mg
Vitamin B_3 (niacin/niacinamide)	50–100 mg
Vitamin B_6 (pyridoxine)	50–100 mg
Vitamin B_{12} (cobalamin)	50–100 mcg
Folic acid	400–800 mcg
Biotin	50–200 mcg
Choline	25–100 mg
Inositol	25–100 mg
PABA	25–100 mg

- *Calcium and magnesium.* Take 500–1,000 milligrams of calcium and 250–500 milligrams of magnesium daily, with 400–1,000 international units of vitamin D if needed. Calcium and magnesium are minerals crucial to many aspects of health, including the cardiovascular system, and also the bones, teeth, and muscles. They work best when taken together because they tend to function synergistically. When you see calcium working in the body, magnesium is usually present. They are natural partners. Their functioning is further optimized by the presence of vitamin D.

Calcium is one of the most important minerals for everyone, especially if you are in your senior years. That's because calcium can be leached from bones and teeth with advancing age—a process called *resorption*. The condition of brittle bones caused by excessive resorption is called *osteoporosis*. But calcium has other important functions in the body. Several studies show that it protects against hypertension and that it might in fact even be more effective than antihypertensive drugs—and free of nasty side effects.

Magnesium, the bodily partner of calcium, is crucial for cardiac functioning because it plays such an important role in regulating the heart's rhythm. Magnesium also helps to lower blood pressure and reduce angina symptoms. However, close to 50 percent of people with cardiovascular problems are deficient in magnesium, perhaps because some of the diuretic pills prescribed for blood pressure tend to leach magnesium from the body. Also, the typical American diet tends to be deficient in magnesium.

Magnesium is also important for adenosine triphosphate (ATP) metabolism. Remember that this is a crucial compound necessary for the conversion of glucose into energy. Magnesium deficiency can result in increased insulin resistance and, ultimately, in diabetes. One study, published in the medical journal *Circulation,* supported the use of oral magnesium therapy to improve endothelial function and exercise tolerance in people with coronary artery disease.

Since calcium and magnesium work together and should be taken together, they are available in calcium-magnesium combination tablets. The optimum ratio of calcium to magnesium is 2:1 (two parts calcium to one part magnesium). Studies have also suggested that vitamin D is necessary to facilitate the functioning of calcium and magnesium, and thus the relationship is a triad. Some supplements are now available that contain not only a correct balance of calcium and magnesium but also some additional vitamin D. If you can't find one of these, then just take a calcium and magnesium product and try to supplement with your own vitamin D—particularly if you do not get many opportunities to go outdoors. (Sunlight is necessary to help our bodies manufacture vitamin D.) Or take your calcium and magnesium together with your multivitamin and mineral supplement, which contains vitamin D.

Who should take calcium and magnesium? Anyone over the age of sixty and all postmenopausal women should take supplemental calcium to protect the bones and teeth. It is never too late to start calcium supplementation and you should definitely do so, even if osteoporosis has already set in. Calcium and magnesium will also help individuals with hypertension, coronary artery disease, or arrhythmia, as well as those who suffer from insulin resistance or diabetes.

Note: Normal quantities of calcium, magnesium, and vitamin D should have no adverse effects. However, taking extremely high doses of calcium (more than 2,500 milligrams a day) can result in a condition called *hypercalcemia,* or elevated calcium levels in the blood. There is no risk of developing this dangerous condition if you keep your calcium supplementation to the recommended dosages. The same is true for vitamin D. Overdoses can be dangerous, but a normal intake has no known side effects. A few of my patients have reported loose bowels or diarrhea with high doses of magnesium, but these symptoms clear up completely when the dosage is reduced or the supplement is discontinued.

- *Essential fatty acids.* Take 2,000–6,000 mg daily. Earlier, we discussed the role of essential fatty acids (EFAs) at length. Now we will look at the use of EFAs in supplement form, specifically to reduce LDL and triglyceride levels, to enhance HDL levels, and for their other benefits. Aside from lowering cholesterol, these compounds also improve the elasticity of the arterial walls, serve as blood thinners, and may even have some anti-inflammatory properties. Additionally, they have been shown to reduce restenosis following angioplasty procedures.

    The best type of EFA supplement to take is one that contains both EPA and DHA. Typically, fish-oil capsules contain 1,000 milligrams of oil, with 180 milligrams of EPA and 120 milligrams of DHA and about 700 milligrams of other oils. Be sure to buy only the highest-quality fish oil supplements you can find, to be sure that the manufacturer tests for the presence of heavy metals such as mercury and for by-products of oxidation. After you have opened the bottle, it is best to store it in the refrigerator because fish oil spoils easily. Many fish-oil preparations contain small amounts of vitamin E, which protects them from oxidizing, the chemical process responsible for spoilage.

Who should take essential fatty acid supplements? People with elevated triglycerides, elevated fibrinogen, elevated cardiac CRP, or low HDL cholesterol levels are excellent candidates for EFA supplementation. If you have undergone balloon angioplasty or bypass surgery, EFA supplements are extremely important components of successful recovery.

Note: Some people report an unpleasant fishy taste or "fish burps" after using fish-oil supplements. This can sometimes be addressed by changing to a supplement manufactured by a different company. In rare cases, EFA supplements may contribute to loose bowels. Reducing the dosage might help if you encounter this problem. Finally, as with vitamin E, you should stop taking EPA products prior to any surgical procedures you might be having, because they serve as blood thinners.

Level 3: Moderate-Risk Program

As risk factors increase, additional supplementation becomes necessary. Some supplements overlap with the level 1 and level 2 programs and apply to everyone in higher risk categories, and you can find a complete description of these earlier in the chapter. There are also other supplements that you should add depending on the *cause* of your elevated risk.

- *Multivitamin and mineral complex* (see table 12.1).
- *Vitamin C.* Take 1,000–2,000 mg daily.
- *Vitamin E.* Take a supplement supplying 400–800 IU of mixed tocopherols and 50–200 mg of tocotrienols daily.

- *Vitamin B-complex with folic acid.* Take a supplement that supplies 100–200 mg of vitamin B_6, 1,000–5,000 mcg of vitamin B_{12}, and 800–5,000 mcg of folic acid daily. In addition to the basic B-complex supplement, you need more vitamin B_6, vitamin B_{12}, and folic acid, as well as niacin, which will be discussed separately below. These are the members of the B group most closely associated with cholesterol and homocysteine reduction and with other cardiovascular benefits.
- *Calcium and magnesium.* Take 800–1,600 mg of calcium and 400–800 mg of magnesium each day, with 400–1,000 IU of vitamin D if necessary.
- *Essential fatty acids.* Take 3,000–6,000 mg a day.
- *Niacin.* Take 500–2,000 mg daily, taken in divided doses, and *always* with a meal. This B vitamin can play an enormous role in cholesterol reduction, and there is a vast amount of scientific research devoted to it. You will often see two names for vitamin B_3: *niacin* and *niacinamide.* Niacin has the most cardiac protective effects. Niacinamide has a less powerful impact on such cardiovascular factors as high cholesterol, but it is quite helpful in promoting relaxation, reducing anxiety, and slowing the progress of degenerative arthritis.

Niacin is a very potent agent for lowering LDL ("bad") cholesterol and triglycerides. It appears to have two major mechanisms of action. First of all, it blocks the liver's production of VLDL (very-low-density lipoprotein). Remember that this is an important component of the triglyceride "package" that travels through the bloodstream. Without VLDL, triglycerides cannot be transported. When the liver reduces its production of VLDL, it results in lower blood levels of triglycerides. Niacin has also been shown to actually raise levels of HDL ("good") cholesterol, further promoting general cardiovascular health.

Niacin also appears to reduce the impact of a prostaglandin called PGI_2. Prostaglandins are hormone-like substances produced by our cells. Like hormones, they stimulate target cells into action. Unlike hormones, however, they act locally, near the sites where they are synthesized, instead of being manufactured in a gland and discharging their mission elsewhere in the body. Derivatives of fatty acids, prostaglandins regulate all our bodily functions, including those of the cardiovascular, immune, nervous, and reproductive systems.

There are numerous prostaglandins that perform different and often opposing sets of functions. The key is for them to be in balance with one another. For example, there are a series of anti-inflammatory prostaglandins and another series of pro-inflammatory prostaglandins. As long as both are present in the correct quantities, they are part of the body's checks-and-balances system that creates just the right amount of inflammation when necessary and quells the inflammation when the job has been done.

The prostaglandins involved in blood clotting are another example. As we have mentioned so many times, we need blood clots in order to survive. There is a substance called *thromboxane A_2* (TXA_2) that promotes blood clotting and the narrowing of vascular smooth muscle. It is supposed to be balanced out by a prostaglandin called *prostaglandin I_2* (PGI_2), which is responsible for opposing and balancing out the action of TXA_2 and making sure that no excess clotting or narrowing occurs. Under ordinary circumstances, these two compounds engage in what is called a *cross-discussion* so as to maintain homeostasis, or balance, in the bloodstream. Malfunction of the PGI_2-signaling mechanism can lead to excessive blood clotting and narrowing of the blood vessels.

Interestingly, a group of researchers at University College in Dublin, Ireland, discovered that naturally occurring compounds produced in the course of cholesterol metabolism are actually necessary for normal PGI_2 signaling. The researchers discovered that statin drugs, which inhibit cholesterol formation, also disrupt the normal signaling process of the PGI_2 receptors, which in turn disrupts normal homeostasis in the veins and arteries. This may be why niacin supplementation is especially important for individuals who take statin drugs.

The dual action of niacin—inhibiting cholesterol formation and promoting PGI_2—is a crucial partnership because lowering cholesterol levels can potentially impede the functioning of PGI_2. Increasing the amount of this prostaglandin strengthens its signaling capacity and regulates the balance of clotting and anticlotting factors in the bloodstream.

The safety of niacin supplementation for people with diabetes has been called into question. However, concerns have recently been allayed in a series of studies that have shown niacin to have significant beneficial effects on lipid levels regardless of whether the person had diabetes, and no adverse effects among those with diabetes.

Finally, a word about niacin supplementation and statin therapy: If you are taking a statin drug, niacin supplementation is crucial, because it can help to offset some of the negative effects of these drugs.

Who should take niacin? If you are in the level 3 (moderate-risk) or level 4 (high-risk) category due to elevated LDL, elevated triglyceride levels, or low HDL, you should be taking niacin. You should also take niacin if you are using a statin drug.

Note: Niacin can have some negative effects, including skin flushing and an irritating rash. These symptoms can be mitigated by taking an aspirin or a supplement containing EPA prior to taking the niacin. Some people also experience nausea and other forms of stomach distress. Most experience relief from these symptoms by using a product called *inositol hexanicotinate* (flush-free niacin), in which the niacin compound is bound to inositol, another B vitamin. When you start using niacin, start slowly and gradually increase the dosage to the

- *Arginine.* Take 2,000–6,000 mg daily. Also called L-arginine, this amino acid's primary function is to lower blood pressure. It does this by stimulating the production of nitric oxide, a naturally occurring vasodilator. Remember that this compound is an essential component of endothelial derived relaxing factor (EDRF), which relaxes the endothelium and, indeed, the entire arterial wall. Of course, this reduces the level of pressure in the blood vessels, thereby improving blood pressure. It also improves general endothelial function. A relaxed endothelium is less taut and stretched, so the tiny openings between its cells are smaller. This provides less of an invitation to invading LDL cholesterol cells and plays an important role in preventing the vicious inflammatory cycle discussed earlier. Arginine also has demonstrated impressive effects for both the short term (as soon as two hours) and the long term.

    Who should take arginine? If you suffer from hypertension, angina, peripheral artery disease, inflammation, elevated CRP, or high cholesterol, you should add arginine to your list of supplements.

    Note: Individuals with a history of genital or oral herpes (cold sores) must take arginine with caution, since there have been some reports that taking high doses of arginine can trigger outbreaks.

- *Coenzyme Q_{10}.* Take 150–360 mg daily. Also called *ubiquinone,* this substance has been the subject of increasing research and attention in recent years. Coenzyme Q_{10} is a fat-soluble molecule that is synthesized from cholesterol. It is a coenzyme, which means that it is essential to the normal functioning of enzymes in the body. It is called coenzyme Q_{10} because it consists of a group of compounds called *quinones* and ten units of another compound called *isoprenyl.* It is called *ubiquinone* because it seems to be ubiquitous—it is found in every single cell throughout the body. It resides in the cells' mitochondria, which is the site where cellular energy is produced.

Coenzyme Q_{10} is found in large concentrations in heart muscle because the heart requires a great deal of energy to function effectively. This has led scientists to research the possibility that coenzyme Q_{10} supplementation might have a positive effect on cardiovascular function, and many clinical studies indeed support this contention. Coenzyme Q_{10} supplements have been found to bring improvements in the cardiac function of people with congestive heart failure and angina. It helps to stabilize cardiac membranes responsible for the heart's electrical conduction system, thereby preventing or rectifying arrhythmias. People treated with coenzyme Q_{10} prior to bypass surgery have been found to have better surgical outcomes than those who do not receive this type of supplementation. In addition, coenzyme Q_{10} is an antioxidant in its own right. It works synergistically with other antioxidants, yielding a more powerful process. It has even been successful in reducing high blood pressure. And here's a nice little benefit: Coenzyme Q_{10} has been associated with healing of periodontal disease. Remember that gum disease can contribute to the inflammatory process.

Levels of coenzyme Q_{10} tend to drop with advancing age, so you may need to take higher doses as you get older. Additionally, if you are taking or have ever taken statin drugs, your concentrations of coenzyme Q_{10} could be lower in your bloodstream and heart muscles, so it is especially important for you to use this supplement. Some consumer groups are advocating for a warning to be put on the label of statin drugs, informing consumers that they must supplement with coenzyme Q_{10} if they are using these medications. It is possible that some pharmaceutical companies may create a formula that introduces coenzyme Q_{10} to statin drugs to offset this problem.

Who should take coenzyme Q_{10}? You should take coenzyme Q_{10} if you are taking statin drugs, if you are over the age of sixty, and if you suffer from hypertension, elevated cholesterol, angina, congestive heart failure, gingivitis (gum disease), inflammation, and/or elevated C-reactive protein levels.

Note: There have been a few reports of gastrointestinal upset (loss of appetite, nausea, and diarrhea) associated with extremely high doses of coenzyme Q_{10}. It is best not to use doses over 600 milligrams without the supervision of a health-care provider.

- *Guggulipid (Commiphora mukul).* Take 25–100 mg daily. Although guggulipid is an ancient product, it has been brought to modern Western scientific attention only during the past two decades or so. In India, however, it has been studied for forty years for its use in cholesterol reduction, and Indian health authorities have approved its sale for the treatment of heart disease. In fact, more than 300 tons are used annually for medical purposes in India.

  Guggulipid is an Ayurvedic herb that has shown much promise in addressing elevated cholesterol levels and other cardiovascular problems. (Ayurveda is a traditional Indian system of healing.) The guggul is a spiny shrub or small tree with many branches that is found in the dry, rocky areas of India. Also known as gum-guggul, salai tree, or Indian bedellium, the resin in this plant has been used for centuries to treat a variety of ailments, including thyroid disorders, arthritis, and gum disease. For our purposes, it has been associated with the regulation of serum cholesterol and triglycerides, helping to bring about the desired balance between HDL and LDL. It also helps to clear the liver of LDL accumulations. Best of all, it has no known side effects or problematic drug interactions.

  Although scientists are not sure exactly what the mechanism of action is, they theorize that the impact of guggulipid on cholesterol derives from its ability to metabolize thyroid hormone. Apparently, serum cholesterol levels are reduced by levels of circulating thyroid hormones, and guggulipid stimulates the production of these hormones. Another theory suggests that guggul helps the liver to increase the uptake of the proteins that carry VLDL and LDL cholesterol. This way, serum triglycerides and cholesterol have no transport mechanism and must be excreted. Finally, it is possible that guggul contains a compound that blocks the action of a type of cell receptor called the farnesoid X receptor (FXR), which modulates cholesterol levels. The FXR receptors control cholesterol by regulating the level of bile acids in the body—remember that these are cholesterol-containing fluids secreted by the liver. When the receptors are blocked, the cholesterol in bile has no place to go, so it must be excreted by the system.

Who should take guggulipid? If you have elevated LDL and triglyceride levels and low HDL levels, this herb can be very helpful.

- *Policosanol.* Take 10–20 mg daily. This is a mixture of saturated alcohol compounds derived from the waxes of plants such as sugar cane, rice bran, and soybeans. The majority of policosanol products come from sugar cane, and these have also been the most widely studied. Policosanol is a purified mixture of molecules known as *long-chain alcohols*—alcohols that have no intoxicating effects.

  It appears that policosanol works through several mechanisms. It inhibits the production of cholesterol in the liver, although scientists are still discussing how this process takes place. It is clear that the process involves the notorious HMG-CoA reductase, the enzyme that produces cholesterol and is inhibited by statin drugs. However, it appears that policosanol's mechanism of action is different from that of the statin drugs. One theory is that it interferes with cholesterol synthesis by jumping into the biochemical pathways that *precede* the manufacture of HMG-CoA reductase. This means it interferes with cholesterol production at an even earlier stage than statin drugs do. Another is that it has a gentler, less competitive inhibitory effect directly on HMG-CoA reductase. Whatever its mechanism, policosanol clearly works directly in the liver to reduce the quantity of cholesterol produced.

Policosanol has another benefit, one that is understood. It promotes the process of LDL cholesterol binding, update, and degradation. This means that the cholesterol exiting the liver is more rapidly processed, metabolized, and excreted by the body, which leaves less circulating in the bloodstream. The lower the blood cholesterol levels, the less opportunity for the insidious atherosclerotic drama to play out.

Studies of policosanol have been quite promising. In fact, there are more than fourteen double-blind placebo-controlled studies that indicate a beneficial effect in lowering total cholesterol, LDL, and triglycerides. And of the thirteen trials that measured HDL cholesterol levels, six showed significant increases in HDL following treatment. Few of the subjects in these studies experienced any negative side effects.

Policosanol's effectiveness in reducing cholesterol makes it a viable alternative to statin drugs, but that's not all. This fascinating substance combats other cardiovascular risk factors, including LDL oxidation, platelet aggregation, endothelial cell damage, and smooth muscle proliferation, and has been shown to be helpful for people with intermittent claudication.

Who should take policosanol? I recommend this supplement to people in the moderate-risk and high-risk groups, especially if they have elevated LDL cholesterol levels and/or low HDL levels. Since there is virtually no downside to using this product, I suggest you take it if you have other problems as well, including inflammation and elevated CRP levels.

- *Red yeast rice.* Take 1,200–2,400 mg daily. This has been both a food and medicinal agent in China since the Tang dynasty in the year 800. However, the active constituents were not discovered by modern Western scientists until the late 1970s. This traditional Chinese food results from adding a purple-colored yeast organism called *Monascus purpureus* to steamed rice and then fermenting the mixture.

To call red yeast rice an alternative to statin drugs is not quite accurate because, actually, red yeast rice contains naturally occurring statins. What is alternative about it is that, according to several major studies, it manages to lower cholesterol as much as prescription statin drugs but without the negative side effects. It is consumed in large quantities in many East Asian countries. Japan is the world's main consumer. In fact, it was in Japan that scientists first isolated the principal active ingredient in red yeast rice, a statin called *monacolin K*. Since then, nine additional statins of the monacolin class have been identified in this ancient food product. All of them are antioxidants, but that is not the primary mechanism of action. More important, they all inhibit the action of HMG-CoA reductase.

Red yeast rice has additional benefits not found in synthetic statin drugs. These benefits derive from the fact that this amazing plant compound contains numerous sterols (beta-sitosterol, campesterol, stigmasterol, and sapogenin), isoflavones, and monounsaturated fatty acids that may all play a significant role in reducing cholesterol levels. For this reason, red yeast rice probably lowers cholesterol through multiple mechanisms, not only through the inhibition of HMG-CoA reductase. The presence of other monacolins, as well as the presence of other phytocompounds, may be the reason that smaller quantities of red yeast rice are necessary to bring about significant cholesterol reduction as compared with statin drugs. The typical daily dosage of 2,400 milligrams of red yeast rice is equivalent to a dosage of 4.8 milligrams of lovastatin, yet the dosage of lovastatin used in clinical trials is typically 20 to 40 milligrams per day, a dosage far greater than what is typically used to gain similar benefits evidenced with red yeast rice. As a result, it is unlikely that the beneficial effects achieved with red yeast rice are solely the result of the lovastatin content of the supplement and are more likely due to the other compounds that contribute to its cholesterol-lowering effect.

Scientists theorize that red yeast rice not only inhibits the formation of cholesterol in the liver (which is what statin drugs do) but also serves as an antioxidant, preventing the oxidation of cholesterol in the bloodstream and thereby reducing its accumulation along the arterial walls. Some additional compounds in red yeast rice have been found to inhibit cholesterol absorption in the intestine.

Why is red yeast rice such a well-kept secret? I believe there are two reasons. One is that some cardiologists are uninformed about natural products and are therefore distrustful of them. One of my patients, who had extremely high cholesterol levels, told me that he asked his cardiologist about using red yeast rice as an alternative to lovastatin for cholesterol reduction. "Oh, the stuff definitely works," his doctor answered. "But you know that with these herbs, we really don't know how much of the active ingredient you'll be getting. But with a drugs we can measure the exact dosage."

I disagree with this doctor. As you will see below, it is possible to recommend a dosage of an herb or natural supplement, just as it is possible to prescribe a specific dosage of a pharmaceutical drug. Of course, you will need to follow the guidelines earlier in this chapter and use a high-quality and reliable brand. In the case of red yeast rice, as in the case of other natural supplements and botanicals, make sure you buy a standardized product to ensure the quality of the active ingredients. If you do this, there is no reason you cannot follow a program as rigorous and individualized as the one emanating from the doctor's prescription pad.

The second reason that red yeast rice has not become as accepted as it could be is that in late 2001, the FDA banned one formulation of the product because of its high statin content. According to the FDA, the medicinal qualities contained in red yeast rice were so great that it had to be considered a prescription drug rather than a food supplement. The ruling was specifically directed at a company called Pharmanex, which manufactured a formulation of red yeast rice called Cholestin. Pharmanex appealed the ruling and lost, and so were forced to discontinue sales of Cholestin. The ruling was based on the fact that Pharmanex processed specific strains of red yeast rice to yield unnaturally high levels of lovastatin.

Today, Pharmanex has reformulated its Cholestin product and uses policosanol, derived from honeybee wax, instead of red yeast rice. However, other products with red yeast rice are still available. It appears that the FDA ruling covers only certain standardized red yeast rice extracts, which they consider to be drugs, rather than nutritional supplements. The FDA stipulates that the total lovastatin content of a red yeast rice extract must not exceed 0.26 percent or it will be considered a drug.

Where does this leave the consumer? How can you tell which products to use if they are not standardized? You can purchase red yeast rice at health-food stores and can obtain special formulations designed (within the restrictions imposed by the FDA) to lower cholesterol levels from mail-order companies that manufacture natural products. A list of some recommended sources appears in the Resources section at the end of this book.

Who should take red yeast rice? If you have elevated total cholesterol, LDL cholesterol, triglycerides, or CRP, you should be taking daily red yeast rice supplements.

Note: Human trials have not shown liver enzyme elevation or kidney impairment in people who take between 1,200 and 2,400 milligrams of red yeast rice per day, even though this product contains naturally occurring statins. However, I believe that it is logical to avoid taking red yeast rice if you are pregnant or nursing, or have preexisting liver or kidney impairments. Certainly, if you are taking medications such as niacin, gemfibrozil

(Lopid), cyclosporin (Neoral, Sandimmune), erythromycin (E-Mycin, ERYC, and others), clarithromycin (Biaxin), or protease inhibitors for HIV disease, you should not take red yeast rice except under the supervision of your health-care provider. Some people have reported mild headaches or gastrointestinal discomfort (such as heartburn and gas). If you are using red yeast rice on a long-term basis, I suggest also taking supplemental coenzyme Q_{10} because synthetic HMG-CoA reductase inhibitors reduce the production of coenzyme Q_{10} in the body. Although I have seen no evidence of this with red yeast rice, I feel that supplementation with coenzyme can't hurt and can only be beneficial.

Level 4: High-Risk Program

If you are in the high-risk group, you need to build on the supplements listed for those in the prevention, low-risk, and moderate-risk groups. It may seem as if you will be popping an awful lot of pills during the day, but this is not really so different from the lifestyle of most Americans who have heart disease and/or multiple risk factors, who may be taking cholesterol-lowering drugs and antihypertension drugs, and possibly others, such as anti-inflammatories, insulin, antacids, and/or antidepressants. In fact, I have had meals with people, especially with older adults, who pull out an entire pill bottle of different-sized and colored capsules, and pharmacies continue to sell enormous "weekly pill boxes" to help keep these medications organized.

The good news is that as you improve your health and go *down* to lower levels of risk, you should be able to decrease your use of these supplements to maintenance dosages.

- *Multivitamin and multimineral supplement.* Take as directed on the product label.
- *Vitamin C.* Take 1,000–3,000 mg daily.

- *Vitamin E.* Take 400–800 IU daily.
- *Vitamin B-complex with folic acid.* Take a supplement that supplies 50–100 mg of most of the major B vitamins, as well as 50–100 mg of vitamin B_6, 500–1,000 mcg of vitamin B_{12}, and 400–800 mcg of folic acid daily.
- *Calcium and magnesium.* Take 800–1,600 mg of calcium and 400–800 mg of magnesium daily.
- *Essential fatty acids.* Take 3,000–8,000 mg daily.
- *Niacin.* Take 1,000–3,000 mg daily, in divided doses.
- *Arginine.* Take 2,000–6,000 mg daily.
- *Coenzyme Q_{10}.* Take 200–400 mg daily.
- *Guggulipid.* Take 25–100 mg daily.
- *Policosanol.* Take 10–20 mg daily.
- *Red yeast rice.* Take 1,200–2,400 mg daily.
- *Alpha-lipoic acid.* Take 100–300 mg daily. This is a potent antioxidant that helps to neutralize the harmful effects of free radicals. It enhances the antioxidant activity of vitamins C and E, as well as the enzyme glutathione. It facilitates the conversion of food into energy and is important in maintaining normal blood-sugar levels. This makes it a useful drug for people with diabetes, along with the fact that it helps in preventing and treating diabetic neuropathies. Alpha-lipoic acid also assists the liver in detoxification, supports the nervous system, and helps to provide energy within muscles.

    Who should take alpha-lipoic acid? If you are trying to prevent or treat diabetic neuropathy, suffer from insulin resistance, or have high triglycerides, this supplement can be extremely helpful. Because it supports and promotes the detoxification process in the liver, you should use it if you are taking a statin drug or even a natural alternative to statins, such as red yeast rice and policosanol, or if your liver has been overtaxed by overexposure to environmental toxins, pesticides, or heavy metals.
- *Bromelain.* Take 500–2,000 mg daily. This is an enzyme derived from pineapples. Bromelain has wide applications and can be

especially helpful for inflammation caused by sports injuries and general muscle aches and pains. Its anti-inflammatory effects may help those with elevated CRP levels, since this is a blood marker of inflammation. Bromelain should be taken between meals rather than with meals, because if taken with food, it serves more as a digestive enzyme rather than an anti-inflammatory substance.

Who should take bromelain? Individuals with elevated CRP levels should use this supplement.

- *Ginkgo (Ginkgo biloba).* Take 40–160 mg daily. This supplement is derived from the ginkgo tree, the oldest leaf-bearing tree in North America. This tree can live for as long as one thousand years and grow to the extraordinary height of 122 feet. Perhaps the very health of the tree hints at the health it can confer to those who use ginkgo supplements, which are rich in flavonoid-containing substances.

    Ginkgo has been widely studied for its success in improving circulation in the extremities and in the carotid arteries. This enhances blood flow to the brain, which may be one of the reasons ginkgo has also been associated with improvements in memory and cognitive function. Many studies have suggested that ginkgo confers protective benefits against Alzheimer's disease, possibly through this mechanism, and possibly through its antioxidant properties. Ginkgo has some mild anti-inflammatory and blood-thinning effects and has also been found to be useful for those recovering from a stroke.

    Who should take Ginkgo biloba? The main cardiovascular benefit of ginkgo is facilitation of recovery from stroke. If you have had a stroke, you should certainly take this important supplement. I also advise patients to take it if there is a family history of Alzheimer's disease, or if they wish to improve their memory or mental acuity, even in the absence of cardiac symptoms or risk factors.

Note: Ginkgo can potentiate the action of blood thinners, so if you are taking one of these medications, please check with your health-care provider before using it. And do not take it prior to surgery, again because of potential blood-thinning effects.

- *Garlic.* Take 400–600 mg daily. Garlic is known to be a highly effective cholesterol-buster and blood thinner that also has powerful anti-inflammatory properties. Numerous studies have supported the use of garlic supplements (not just fresh garlic in foods) for cholesterol reduction. Taking garlic supplements is an excellent way to augment your cardiac-care program because you would have to eat large quantities of fresh garlic to obtain the results you get from garlic pills. Many people object to the odor of garlic, but deodorized garlic supplements are available in health-food stores.

    Who should take garlic? If you suffer from high cholesterol, high blood pressure, or inflammation, garlic should help you.

- *Grapeseed extract.* Take 100–200 mg daily. This is a supplement that is very high in a group of flavonoids called *proanthocyanidins,* which have strong antioxidant and anti-inflammatory effects. Grapeseed extract neutralizes free radicals, strengthens capillaries, improves circulation to the extremities, and protects against bruising. It is known to inhibit the process of LDL cholesterol oxidation. You can obtain grapeseed extract in tablet or capsule form in health-food stores.

    Who should take grapeseed extract? If your CRP levels are high, which points to the presence of inflammation in your bloodstream, grapeseed extract should be particularly helpful. If you suffer from angina or intermittent claudication, you might try it as well because it increases circulation to the arms and legs.

- *Hawthorn.* Take 300–600 mg of standardized extract daily. This herb has been approved in Germany and Asia for mild cases of congestive heart failure and cardiac insufficiency (lack of sufficient blood flow to the heart) because it contains a flavonoid that is a vasodilator—a substance that causes blood vessels to relax and dilate, thereby increasing coronary blood flow. In fact, hawthorn has been shown to increase coronary circulation by 20 to 40 percent. Since hawthorn relaxes the walls of blood vessels, it is also useful in bringing down blood pressure levels.

Who should take hawthorn? If you are suffering from congestive heart failure, cardiac insufficiency, or intermittent claudication, then hawthorn might be quite helpful. It can also help to reduce blood pressure.

Note: It is generally recommended that you not take hawthorn if you are taking digitalis (Digoxin) or other drugs in the same category, unless you are being monitored by a physician.

- *L-Carnitine*. Take 500–2,000 mg daily. This substance consists of a molecule of vitamin C linked to lysine, an amino acid. The most important function L-carnitine serves is to burn free fatty acids by bringing them into the mitochondria of cells, where they can be turned into energy. It thus lowers triglyceride levels by whisking away circulating triglycerides and importing them into cells for immediate conversion into fuel.

    L-carnitine also increases blood flow to the heart and lungs, so I recommend it for people with angina and congestive heart failure. In these conditions, the heart muscle is too weak to pump adequate quantities of blood to the lungs. People become tired and weak. In congestive heart failure, fluid surrounds the lungs, making it difficult to talk, breathe, and sleep. By importing triglycerides to the cells of the heart, where they are converted into energy, L-carnitine enables the heart to pump more efficiently and send larger quantities of blood to the lung area. People taking L-carnitine experience improved exercise tolerance and decreased symptoms of angina. Interestingly, L-carnitine also seems to raise levels of HDL cholesterol. And in people who have heart attacks, it appears to protect the tissues of the heart against the process of necrosis.

Who should take L-carnitine? If you have elevated triglycerides, insulin resistance, angina, or congestive heart failure, you should be taking L-carnitine supplements on a regular basis.

- *Milk thistle (Silibum marianum).* Take 150–450 mg of extract standardized to 80 percent silymarin content daily. This herb is known to have a positive impact on liver function. In fact, it is commonly recommended for alcoholics whose livers have been negatively affected by their drinking. But everyone can benefit from milk thistle for additional liver support, especially people with cholesterol problems. Remember that cholesterol is metabolized in the liver. In order for the liver to correctly process fat—especially if there is a fat overload—it must be functioning at its best. Milk thistle helps to maximize the liver's effectiveness. And this supplement works: One study showed that milk thistle both lowered LDL and raised HDL cholesterol. Some studies also suggest that it can counteract the negative effects of medications such as statin drugs.

  Who should take milk thistle? If you are taking statin drugs, or even using red yeast rice or policosanol (both of which perform their main functions in the liver), you should consider taking the additional liver support found in milk thistle. The liver is an important organ for detoxification of the entire body. If you are bombarded by toxins such as alcohol, pesticides, pollutants, and heavy metals, milk thistle will assist your liver in ridding the body of these dangerous substances.

- *Pantethine.* Take 300–900 mg daily. This is an activated form of vitamin B_5 (pantothenic acid). The body quickly converts pantethine into an important substance called *coenzyme A,* which affects many biochemical pathways, including those involved in fat metabolism. Pantethine has been used for the past thirty years in Japan to increase levels of HDL cholesterol. It seems to work by slowing the production of cholesterol in the liver and boosting the rate at which the body metabolizes fats. Pantethine can significantly reduce total cholesterol and LDL while increasing HDL cholesterol. It is also very effective in lowering triglyceride levels.

Who should take pantethine? If you have high total or LDL cholesterol levels, high triglycerides, or low HDL cholesterol levels, pantethine can be quite helpful.

- *Taurine.* Take 500–1,500 mg daily. Taurine is a nonessential amino acid. This means that our body manufactures it from cysteine, one of the other essential, sulfur-containing amino acids. It appears to help balance the sodium and potassium concentration in the heart muscle, thereby increasing the heart's ability to contract properly and maintain a regular and vigorous heartbeat. It can therefore be very useful for people with congestive heart failure. It can also help with certain arrhythmias. A person deficient in taurine may be more susceptible to experiencing irregular heartbeat. Taurine has also been helpful in lowering blood pressure. This may be connected with its function in regulating the sodium-potassium balance, not only in the heart muscle but in other cells as well. And here's an interesting fact: Taurine has been quite helpful in treating macular degeneration, a progressive eye condition that often affects older adults.

    Who should take taurine? If you suffer from hypertension, arrhythmia, angina, or congestive heart failure, taurine can be helpful for you.

    Note: It is best to take taurine together either with a carbohydrate or between meals on an empty stomach. Do not take it together with protein because, as an amino acid, it may compete with the amino acids in the food for absorption and therefore may not be fully absorbed properly.

- *Turmeric (Curcuma longa).* Take 200–1,200 mg daily. Turmeric is well known as a spice. Due to its content of a compound known as curcumin, it also has anti-inflammatory effects and is used commonly for the soreness and achiness associated with arthritis. It can also be effective in reducing inflammation in the bloodstream. You can certainly use this spice in cooking; it is yellowish in color and has a distinctive and delicious flavor. However, if you are in a high-risk category and are using this product more aggressively to reduce inflammation, you need to be more precise.

Who should take turmeric (curcumin)? This supplement is especially important for people with elevated CRP levels, which indicate the presence of inflammation.

Choosing Supplements

Vitamins, herbs, and other supplements come in various forms—tablets, capsules, powder, or liquid extracts. Some people find that one form is more agreeable than another. For example, if you have trouble swallowing pills, a liquid or powder form may be your first choice. In general, liquid extracts tend to be more quickly absorbed but less convenient to transport. So if you are taking a supplement several times a day, you may prefer to take a packet of pills to your office, rather than a series of vials with droppers. The important factors are dosage and ingredients. The label should list clearly what the dosage is and what all of the product's components are. For example, different vitamin E supplements contain different combinations of components.

Apart from the type of formulation, how do you choose among the wide array of products available at health-food stores, pharmacies, even supermarkets? There is a great deal of confusion regarding this. Generally speaking, if you require conventional medication for a health problem, your physician writes out a prescription for a specific drug or recommends an over-the-counter category of drugs such as a decongestant or pain reliever. You know these items are FDA-approved for the purpose for which you are taking them, and you assume that they are safe and effective.

Patients often ask me whether the FDA plays a similar role in assuring the safety and efficacy of natural supplements. The answer is no. The

FDA classifies vitamins and herbal products as nondrug substances called *dietary supplements*. Prior to the early 1990s, these dietary supplements were regulated by the FDA as food substances. However, as the popularity of natural supplements grew, it became apparent that they were being used as therapeutic agents rather than as foods. Initially, the FDA proposed to remove all of these items from the market and reevaluate them, using standards set forth for other therapeutic substances, such as drugs. (In order for a drug to be approved by the FDA, it must go through extensive and rigorous testing procedures until it is shown to have a reasonable margin of safety.)

The FDA's plan to remove supplements from the market was greeted by a great public outcry, leading to a compromise legislation, called the Dietary Supplement Health and Education Act of 1994 (DSHEA). Dietary supplements became defined as oral products that are intended to supplement the diet and contain raw or processed forms of one or more of the following: herbs, vitamins, minerals, amino acids, or other botanical products. These products would no longer come under the jurisdiction of the FDA. However, the DSHEA restricted the statements that manufacturers were allowed to put on product labels. A label can claim that the product contains a particular nutrient ("a good source of vitamin C"). It can make general statements about health, such as "eating fiber reduces your risk of cardiovascular disease." Finally, it can claim to promote some specific area of health ("strengthens the immune system"). What it cannot do is claim to address particular diseases ("treats the common cold"). Further, labels that contain health claims must also indicate that the product has not been approved by the FDA and is not intended to diagnose, treat, or prevent any disease. Additionally, a label must provide certain other types of information—for example, the company must indicate what part of the plant an herbal product comes from.

Thus, the FDA may control what's on the label, but it has no say over the contents of the bottle. The responsibility for this lies in the hands of the manufacturers. However, if a product already in the market turns out to be unsafe, the FDA has the authority to remove it from the market.

So, how do you know which brands are reliable? The answer to this is complicated. It is true that not all supplements are created equal. But because supplement companies know that consumers want to feel confident that the products they buy are authentic, efficacious, and safe, they have taken upon themselves the responsibility for hiring independent agencies to approve supplements that meet a set of predetermined criteria. There are currently four agencies that provide a seal of approval for dietary supplements: the United States Pharmacopoeia (USP), NSF International, ConsumerLab.com, and the Good Housekeeping Institute. These companies look at such issues as the cleanliness of the facility where the product was manufactured; the presence or absence of contaminants, pesticides, or toxins in the product; and whether the label accurately reflects the true nature of the product. So when you purchase a dietary supplement, be sure that you look for a product that carries the certification of one of these agencies.

If you are purchasing herbs, you should also look for a *standardized extract*. This means that the active ingredient in the herb is present in a standardized quantity that is known to be effective.

Even though some supplements may not be perfect, and supplements in general may be subjected to criticism because the FDA does not have jurisdiction over quality control, this does not invalidate the use of herbs and supplements. There are many reliable and high-quality products. The Resources section at the back of this book provides a list of companies whose products I personally recommend. If you have a health-care provider who is familiar with herbs and supplements, ask him or her for recommendations as well. Some physicians suggest specific companies and have favorite brands or formulations.

You can obtain supplements at your local health-food store, although many supermarkets and pharmacies are beginning to carry these natural products as well, and there are also many online providers. However, it is likely that your health-food store will carry a better selection than your supermarket will. This is important because when selecting supplements, it is always best to use the ones with the most natural, rather than synthetic, ingredients. And try to avoid those with sugar, artificial colorings, and preservatives, even if they are manufactured from natural ingredients. Of course, if you have allergies, you should avoid taking supplements with even trace amounts of wheat, soy, corn, eggs, and dairy. You can find out what's in a supplement by reading the label, which should indicate the source of the vitamin, mineral, or herb that is the main ingredient, plus any other ingredients used in the formulation of the product. The Resources section will provide a list of the highest quality, most reliable brands of vitamins and supplements.

Tips for Taking and Storing Supplements

Whether or not you get the most out of the supplements you use depends not only on choosing quality products and determining the correct dosage but also on taking them correctly and storing them properly. Following are a number of tips for taking and storing your supplements:

- Take supplements with a meal, unless otherwise specified in this book or on the product label. Food generally helps to enhance absorption and assimilation and to reduce the possibility of indigestion, which can occur when some supplements are taken on an empty stomach.
- Take supplements with water rather than with other beverages.
- Be aware that, although it is rare, some supplements do not mix well with certain medications. This may be more of a concern with herbs than with vitamins and minerals. Although herbs tend to be much freer of side effects than pharmaceutical products, they are still powerful agents and can sometimes negatively interact with certain drugs. If you have any doubts regarding the safety of a particular supplement, please consult your health-care practitioner. The names of several reference books that contain lists of negative herb-drug interactions are listed in the Resources section of the book.
- Keep your supplements out of extreme heat and away from hu-

midity. Store them in a cool, dark cabinet—*not* the medicine cabinet in your bathroom.
- Keep an eye on the expiration date printed on the bottle or package to ensure that supplements are at their maximum potency.
- If you wish to transfer your supplements to a smaller container for purposes of work or travel, make sure to use a container that is opaque (so that it keeps out the light) and that seals tightly.
- As with any type of medication, keep supplements—even vitamins—in a secure place and out of the reach of children.

A Final Word About Supplements

I hope you are not overwhelmed by all of this information on the wonderful array of helpful natural substances. If you have a limited income and cannot buy all of these supplements (which, sadly, are not covered by most health insurance plans), begin with the basic six (multivitamin and mineral complex, vitamin C, vitamin E, vitamin B-complex, calcium and magnesium, and essential fatty acids) and add as many of the other helpful supplements as you can afford. You can choose which are most important based on your level of risk and on your particular risk factors and primary symptoms.

One more caveat: Just because all of these supplements have cardiovascular benefit does not mean you necessarily have to take all of them, and in the dosages recommended. I have found that many of my patients have been able to take fewer nutrients in lower doses. The many other nutrients they take and the numerous other health-promoting activities they undertake seem to work synergistically. So the more you do, the less you might need.

Diet and supplements are mainstays of the DEAR program, and they are necessary for coronary artery healing. But these are still not enough. The next chapter will focus on exercise, which is an extremely important intervention—and an enjoyable one, too!

13 Exercise: A Great Cholesterol-Buster

A man falls into ill health as a result of not caring to exercise.
— ARISTOTLE

A sedentary lifestyle is one of the most serious risk factors for the development of cardiovascular disease. According to recent estimates, those who are sedentary have almost twice the risk of developing CVD as do those who exercise regularly. Unfortunately, most Americans don't realize this. Statistics about inactivity in this country are alarming. Close to 60 percent of the population leads a sedentary lifestyle. As technology has advanced, the need for physical movement has decreased, and people have responded by relaxing into their newfound freedom from physical activity. Most seriously affected are older adults. Studies show that up to three-quarters of the senior population do not exercise at recommended levels.

Earlier generations of Americans not only ate a healthier diet—low in refined sugar, free of chemicals and pesticides, and high in fiber and vegetables—but also got a lot of physical exercise. Instead of hopping into a car, they walked to and from school, to the market, and to other destinations. There were no televisions, so they did not sit for hours on a couch, staring at a box with moving figures. After-dinner relaxation might have involved taking a stroll. Mothers wheeled their babies about in carriages until they fell asleep. Work, whether inside or outside the home, often involved significant physical activity. Aerobic exercise was thus incorporated into people's lifestyles in a natural way, and they were much healthier as a result.

In contrast, our lifestyles are constructed around speed and efficiency. We love e-mails and faxes because they get information from one place to another instantaneously. We look for products that will accomplish their functions with maximum speed—medications that relieve headache pain faster, for example. The last thing we want is to walk someplace for forty-five minutes when a car could get us there in five to ten.

For those of us who cannot walk to and from our destinations, we must find ways to purposely inject exercise into our daily lives. This chapter will discuss why exercise is important to our health and how you can incorporate it into your lifestyle.

What's So Great About Exercise?

It has been known for centuries that exercise is essential to good health, but only recently have scientists begun to understand why this is the case. Let's look at what happens in the body when you engage in exercise.

AEROBIC EXERCISE

Aerobic exercise involves a steady, rhythmic activity. Examples of aerobic exercise include walking, jogging, running, bicycling, canoeing/rowing, dancing, swimming, jumping rope, hiking, skating, and skiing. Aerobic exercise gets its name because of the role of air, or oxygen, in the process—you are inhaling on a regular basis and using the oxygen you have taken in to release stored energy. When you exercise aerobically, you continuously elevate your pulse for a regular period of time. This moves the entire oxygenation process along at a faster and more efficient rate, resulting in a decrease in LDL cholesterol and triglycerides (which are carried away by the more briskly moving bloodstream) and an increase in HDL cholesterol.

Exercise is also an excellent antidote to inflammation. Because it facilitates efficient and rapid circulation of blood, it removes inflammatory substances before they have a chance to build up along blood vessel walls. It also keeps the walls themselves contracting and expanding more efficiently and regularly. This keeps the blood vessels elastic and toned and helps to reduce high blood pressure. In fact, exercise is one of the most important remedies for hypertension and is a crucial adjunct to any good hypertension reduction program.

Aerobic exercise has an array of other benefits that indirectly help the cardiovascular system. For example, the more you exercise, the more stored fat cells are converted into energy to fuel the extra expenditure of energy you need to run, swim, or do whatever you are doing. This helps with weight reduction. And, since obesity is a risk factor for CVD, the weight loss will indirectly be beneficial to your heart and blood vessels. Exercise also is beneficial for people with diabetes because it stimulates a more efficient use of insulin. And aerobic exercise is a wonderful antidepressant. As we will see in the next chapter, depression is a major risk factor for CVD.

Exercise is a wonderful way of handling anxiety as well. When we are stressed or anxious, our bodies release a series of hormones that prepare us for some intense output of physical activity—the so-called *fight-or-flight response*. Exercise burns off some of that excess energy, giving the cardiovascular system what it expects and what it has been primed for and reducing the strain of chronic stress.

Numerous studies have supported aerobic exercise as a crucial component of any program to reduce cholesterol and increase cardiac health.

STRENGTH-BUILDING EXERCISE

Examples of strength-building, or anaerobic, exercise include weight-lifting and using resistance machines. This type of exercise differs from aerobic exercise because, although it utilizes energy and demands increased oxygen, it does not do so in a sustained way. Think of the difference between lifting weights and jogging. When you lift weights, there is a sudden spurt of energy, then a reprieve, then another spurt. When you walk or jog, there is a regular, consistent utilization of oxygen.

But the fact that this is anaerobic (as opposed to aerobic) exercise does not mean that it isn't valuable or even essential. On the contrary, it is necessary for good health in people of all ages, especially older adults. Muscle strength declines by an average of 15 percent per decade after age fifty, and 30 percent per decade after age seventy. This is usually the result of loss of muscle mass, and, although it affects individuals of both genders, it affects women more than men. The results of the Framingham Disability Study show that 45 percent of women above the age of sixty-five and 65 percent of women above the age of seventy-five cannot lift ten pounds.

Weight training restores muscle mass and prevents further deterioration. Strength training can result in a 25 to 100 percent increase in muscle mass. Increased muscle mass means that you feel stronger. After all, you have more muscles to give you the leverage you need to push, pull, or lift. Remember also that a great deal of glucose metabolism and energy conversion take place within the muscles. The less muscle there is, the less energy is produced. The weaker you feel, the less you will be able to engage in aerobic exercise, which will, in turn, negatively affect your circulation and your heart. It is also known that muscle mass protects against osteoporosis. So strength training has an array of benefits.

It's never too late to begin a weight-training regimen. A case study showed an increase in muscle mass in a man in his nineties! As with aerobic exercise, however, don't try to do this on your own. Allow a coach or trainer to assist you in beginning a program that is appropriate for your age and physical condition.

Here is an important warning to take into your weight-training exercises: It is very important to remember to breathe regularly while lifting weights. Don't hold your breath. Breathe out when lifting the weight and breathe in during muscle relaxation between lifts.

STRETCHING AND CALISTHENICS

We tend to use some muscle groups regularly and to neglect others. Much depends on our lifestyle—if we bicycle regularly, for example, we use a particular set of muscles, but may barely move our upper bodies. If we do gardening or some other form of outdoor work, we may use a particular set of arm and shoulder muscles regularly, but neglect our leg muscles. When you start a new exercise regimen (for example, if you usually walk but then start riding a bicycle), you can strain unused muscles or even stress customarily used muscles by using them differently. Stretching helps to tone the muscles before you begin your heavier exercise. It protects you from injury and soreness and enhances balance and flexibility. And because you are less likely to get a charley horse, you are more likely to continue exercising rather than giving up.

What Do the Studies Say?

In study after study, exercise has been shown to be highly effective as a way of reducing problematic blood lipid levels and generally improving cardiovascular health. For example, the Nurse's Study conducted by the Harvard Medical School at Brigham and Women's Hospital looked at 72,000 women. The study found that women who walked briskly five or more hours a week had a 50 percent lower incidence of heart attack than those who did not. Those who walked briskly for three hours per week had a 40 percent lower incidence. The Multiple Risk Factor Intervention Trial (MRFIT) showed similar results. After following 12,130 middle-aged men for seven years, the researchers found that those who exercised moderately had one-third fewer deaths from all causes (including CVD) than those who were sedentary. (Moderate exercise was defined as at least thirty minutes a day of light- or moderate-intensity activities, such as walking, gardening, or doing home repairs.) Interestingly, those who engaged in intense activity did not have significantly lower mortality rates than those who engaged in moderate activity.

Here is another interesting finding, and one that dispels a common myth. Some research has suggested that formerly sedentary seniors who become regularly involved in exercise for the first time in their lives have a lower incidence of CVD than seniors who had been extremely active in their youth but had become sedentary in their older years. The message is clear: Contrary to popular belief, it is never too late to start exercising. And you can't stock up on exercise, resting on the laurels of your former physical fitness and relying upon it to protect you in older years. Pointing nostalgically to yourself in a football uniform during your high school years may boost the ego, but it does nothing to boost your health today. It would be better to put away the photographs and start exercising.

Another popular myth is that for exercise to be helpful, it must be extremely intense and taxing. This myth has been dispelled by several studies. In one study, researchers followed 12,224 healthy men and 3,120 healthy women over an eight-year period. Participants were divided into five groups, ranging from the least fit to the most fit. At the end of the study, the participants in the first group (the least fit and most sedentary) had a death rate more than three times greater than those in the fifth group (the most fit and least sedentary). Again, an interesting finding was that those in the second, third, and fourth groups (who engaged in less activity than those in the fifth) still had a dramatically lower mortality rate than those in the most sedentary group. The implications are clear: Engaging in regular aerobic exercise, even low-intensity activities, offers major protection against all forms of illness, including CVD.

This is important information because many people believe that they must plunge into a grueling exercise regimen to rectify damage done by years of poor eating habits and a sedentary existence. This is untrue and dangerous. For a sedentary person to start a running program without a period of gradual breaking-in can be hazardous. Newspapers often carry reports of overweight, out-of-shape people who collapse while jogging or shoveling snow. Don't overdo it. Engage in aerobic activity that challenges but does not overstrain. To do this, you may have to shed a common belief about exercise—"no pain, no gain." It is not necessary to push your body to its limits to gain the cardiovascular benefits of exercise. In fact, it is detrimental to do so.

A Sensible Plan

As we have seen, care of the body is one of the most important activities you can engage in, but for some reason it is associated with some of the least sensible behaviors, especially in the United States. Following is a safe exercise plan that takes your history, risk profile, and lifestyle into account.

SEE YOUR DOCTOR

If you are over the age of thirty-five and want to start an exercise program, you should begin by talking to your health-care provider, especially if you have a history of high blood pressure or CVD. You may be asked to take a stress test that monitors your blood pressure and heart rhythm while you are walking on a treadmill. This will provide your doctor with important information about the safety of your proposed exercise program. Your doctor might order certain blood tests, including a lipid profile, serum chemistry, and complete blood count. If you have any cardiac difficulties, such as certain types of arrhythmias, you may need to modify your program or work with a specialized exercise therapist or trainer.

EXAMINE YOUR LIFESTYLE

Many people begin and quickly abandon exercise programs because they have not realistically assessed their lifestyle and the type of exercise regimen that they can sustain over a long-term period. I like to divide exercise into two categories—cheap and easy, and high-maintenance—as follows:

- Cheap and easy: aerobics, bicycle riding, climbing stairs, dancing, jogging, jumping rope, running in place, stretching, walking.
- High-maintenance: manual labor, mountain climbing/hiking, shoveling snow, skating, skiing (cross-country and downhill), snowmobiling, swimming, tennis.

I call the first category cheap and easy because you don't have to do much or go far in order to engage in these activities. You don't have to go to a swimming pool or belong to a health club. You can walk, run, dance, jump rope, or climb stairs in your own home or on your local streets for free.

So if you have several hours a week to devote exclusively to exercise, you might choose a high-maintenance activity such as swimming or skating, which requires a specialized setting or equipment. But if you have only three twenty-minute slots each week, then walking picks itself as the lowest maintenance activity, therefore the easiest to sustain. Walking can also be fit into the nooks and crannies of a busy schedule. On a long phone call? Pace to and fro, or go up and down the staircase. You would be surprised how much ground you can cover. (And if it's an upsetting conversation, the exercise will help take the edge off the anxiety as well.) Do you need milk from the convenience store? You can get twenty minutes of exercise simply by biking there and back. These low-maintenance exercises are ideal for individuals with demanding family obligations and anyone whose lifestyle leaves too little space for planned blocks of specially designated exercise time.

But don't leave fun out of the picture. If exercise becomes boring—

something you dread—then you are less likely to stay with it. Choose an exercise you enjoy or try to make it fun. Consider walking together with your spouse or a friend. Walking can be a wonderful bonding experience. Or take a portable stereo and play your favorite music or listen to an interesting audiotape. You may end up looking forward to your daily walk or jog—or even find yourself adding extra minutes!

If it is difficult for you to break ingrained habits, consider ways to incorporate exercise into these established routines. For example, you can move the treadmill or stationary bicycle in front of the television or into the kitchen. That way you can watch television or do the dishes while exercising.

START SLOWLY AND KEEP BUILDING UP

Once you have decided on a particular form of exercise, it's time to start incorporating it into your life. If you have been sedentary for many years, you would be well advised to start slowly, especially if you are an older adult. Walk to the mailbox to get the mail instead of asking someone else to do this for you. Walk to work instead of using a taxi, bus, or subway. Get off the couch to change the television channel instead of using the remote control. If you play golf, walk from one hole to the next instead of using a golf cart. Take the stairs instead of the elevator. Use every opportunity to begin moving your body and let increased dexterity be your guide and your goal. These opportunities will arise daily, but not necessarily on an organized or planned basis. It is important to be proactive in creating an exercise regimen. Here are a few examples of ways for those who have not been physically active to begin:

- Begin walking five minutes a day three times a week, then gradually work your way up to twenty minutes a day five days a week. Start by walking at a slow pace, then gradually increase.
- Purchase a treadmill or stationary bicycle and begin with the lowest intensity settings for five minutes a day three times a

week. Work yourself up to longer periods of time and more challenging settings as your physical stamina increases.
- Join a health club and begin using the swimming pool. You may need to spend the first weeks simply moving your limbs around in the water, acquainting yourself with the feeling of being underwater and reacquainting yourself with your body parts. Eventually, you can begin to do a low-intensity stroke, such as the breaststroke, for five minutes, three times a week. You can gradually increase the amount of time, as well as the intensity.

The ultimate goal is to reach your personal intensity maximum. One way to assess this is to look at the maximum intensity you can sustain while simultaneously carrying on a conversation. Sometimes, this is called the *talk test*. Another test of intensity involves measuring your pulse rate and comparing it to the figures in table 13.1. Your target is to reach a pulse rate that is consistent with your age and physical condition, and to sustain that during your exercise.

Finally, be aware of warning signs. If your muscles or joints feel sore after you have exercised, you may have overdone it, but there is no need to worry; just cut back until you can work up to a higher intensity without pain. But if you experience chest pain or pressure, trouble breathing or shortness of breath, lightheadedness, wooziness, dizziness, difficulty keeping your balance, or acute nausea, stop what you are doing immediately and call your doctor.

TABLE 13.1
Target Pulse Rates by Age

Use this table to help determine your target exercising pulse rate. Note that for each age, a range of pulse rates is provided. Also, be aware that if you are taking prescription medication, especially one that may affect your heart rate, your target zone may be less than the figures in this table. Beta-blockers such as metoprolol (Lopressor)

(continued)

and propranolol (Inderal), for example, are known to affect heart rate. Check with your doctor to find the ideal target zone for you.

Age	Minimum Rate	Maximum Rate
25	136	156
30	133	152
35	130	148
40	126	144
45	122	140
50	119	136
55	115	132
60	112	128
65	108	124
70	105	120
75	101	116
80	98	112

To determine your pulse rate, do the following:

1. Lightly place two fingertips on your carotid artery (the main artery in the side of your neck, just below the ear).
2. Count your pulse for fifteen seconds, beginning with 0.
3. Multiply that number by 4.

This will give you your pulse rate per minute.

Finally, remember that the intensity of exercise is a subjective thing. A brisk walk may be challenging for some but not for others. Some people can jog slowly and like to use their morning run as a social time. Others find even a slow jog to be quite taxing. For this reason, I have divided some of the suggested exercises in the exercise pyramids at the end of this chapter into two categories: low-intensity and high-intensity. You can choose whichever you prefer.

STRETCH BEFORE YOU EXERCISE

Stretching is essential for avoiding injury and muscle cramps. It increases your flexibility and range of motion, strengthens a weak back, and alleviates lower back pain. To help reduce your risk of injury or discomforts such as shin splints, it is a good idea to stretch for five to ten minutes both before and after strenuous exercise.

When you stretch, remember to breathe deeply and to try to hold each position for a minimum of five seconds. Eventually you can work your way up to thirty seconds. Repeat each stretch at least three times. Never force a muscle. Stretching should be done slowly and gently. And when you stretch, maintain each position until you feel a gentle pulling—do not bounce. If you have had any recent surgery or have muscle or joint problems, consult your physician or health-care provider before embarking upon a stretching program.

WARM UP AND COOL DOWN

Don't just jump into the most intensive peak of your exercises. Begin with warm-ups, which should consist of some stretching, as well as slower versions of what you are planning to do. For example, you can begin your jog by walking for a few minutes, then gradually accelerating your pace until you are jogging. Likewise, don't suddenly stop exercising when you are at the peak of intensity. Slow your pace and allow a few minutes to cool down.

BE CREATIVE ABOUT YOUR PROGRAM

For busy people, incorporating exercise into your schedule can be as challenging as the physical exertion of the exercise itself. It is important for you to look at your own life and figure out ways to include a regular exercise regimen. You can combine aerobic and anaerobic exercise by attaching weights to your ankles and wrists when you walk. There are Velcro versions of these bracelets available that enable you to progressively increase the heaviness you are carrying. You can also hold increasingly heavy weights in your hands as you walk. Some workout machines offer one-stop shopping when it comes to exercise, combining aerobic and strength-building exercises in a single piece of equipment. If you are committed to your exercise program, you will find many ways to implement that commitment.

ADDITIONAL EXERCISE TIPS

Many people who start exercising for the first time end up developing unhealthy exercise habits. This can end up sabotaging even the best-intentioned efforts. If you are new to exercise, you may not be familiar with some of the things that experienced exercisers know. Here are some tips to help you start off on the right foot:

- Wear loose, comfortable clothing.
- Wear shoes that fit well and have a good arch support and an elevated, cushioned heel to absorb shock.
- Do not hold your breath during exercise.
- Move in slow, controlled motions rather than fast, jerky motions.
- Tune in to radio reports regarding heat and air-pollution levels if you plan to exercise outdoors. If conditions are not conducive to healthy outdoor exercise, consider using an indoor facility, such as a gym, track, or shopping mall (many malls are open before and after hours for walkers).
- If you are walking outdoors, be sure to wear a head covering and sunglasses to protect you from the sun's damaging rays.
- Carry bottled water with you and drink frequently so you don't get dehydrated.

- If you have difficulties with balance, investigate devices to increase your safety.
- Try to exercise with a friend—it makes exercise both safer and more enjoyable.

Customizing Your Exercise Program

As in the area of diet, it is useful to look at appropriate exercise programs in terms of four cardiovascular risk categories, with an exercise pyramid for each. Remember that as you become healthier, your level of risk will (hopefully) decrease. You can then adjust your exercise program accordingly. Following are specific exercise recommendations for each level.

LEVEL 1: PREVENTION

If your risk factors are negligible to very low, this activity program should suit your needs. You need to stretch on a regular basis so as to maintain flexibility and suppleness, but you do not need to do more than twenty to thirty minutes of aerobic exercise each day, depending on your choice of low-intensity versus high-intensity exercises. Of course, you can combine both types of exercise (ten minutes of walking and twenty of jogging) in a single day, or you can alternate different types of exercises on a weekly basis.

If you enjoy competitive sports, feel free to continue engaging in them, but don't regard them as a substitute for aerobic exercise. Most competitive sports (except for marathon running) involve a great deal of stop-and-go. For example, in softball, you stand on base while the opposing team is up at bat and then have four furious seconds activity as you tag an opponent who is trying to slide into second; in tennis, you chase the ball, then stand, then run again in short spurts. Aerobic exercise requires a consistent, steady output of energy.

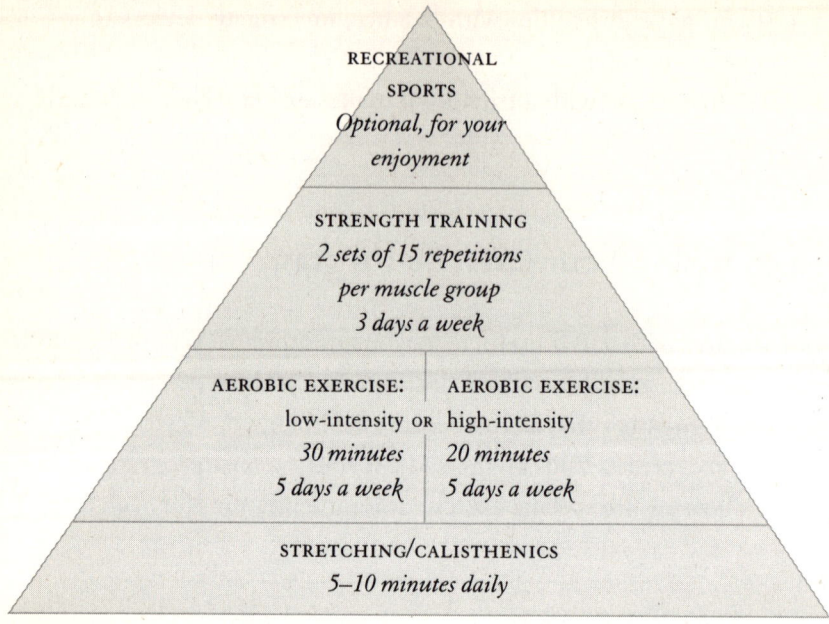

Figure 13.1 The Prevention Exercise Pyramid
The figure above illustrates the amounts of different types of exercise recommended for people in risk category level 1 (prevention).

LEVEL 2: THE MILD RISK

You need to be somewhat more aggressive in your approach to exercise, just as you were in your approach to diet. Your program is almost identical to that for level 1 (prevention), with one exception—you need to add ten minutes to your aerobic exercise, regardless of whether you are engaging in low-intensity or high-intensity activities.

Exercise: A Great Cholesterol-Buster

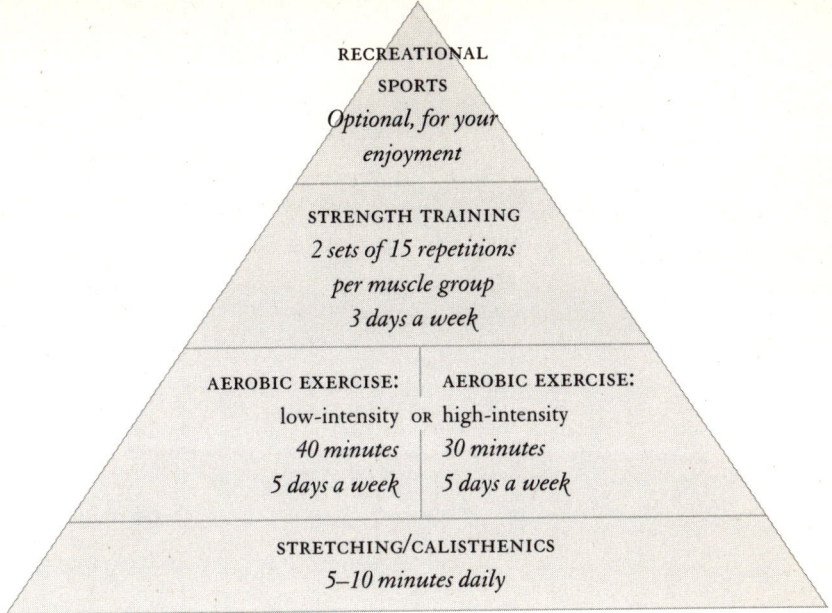

Figure 13.2 The Mild-Risk Exercise Pyramid
The figure above illustrates the amounts of different types of exercise recommended for people in risk category level 2 (mild risk).

LEVEL 3: MODERATE RISK

You have to be even more aggressive than those in the moderate-risk category. You also have to be more careful. I would advise you to eliminate recreational sports until your risk level has decreased because their stop-and-go nature strains the heart. Once your risk level is reduced, your heart should be able to withstand the extra stress caused by sudden spurts of activity followed by a period of inactivity, but you need to be in better shape and preferably to have the approval of your doctor. You also need to increase your aerobic exercise by engaging in it on a daily basis.

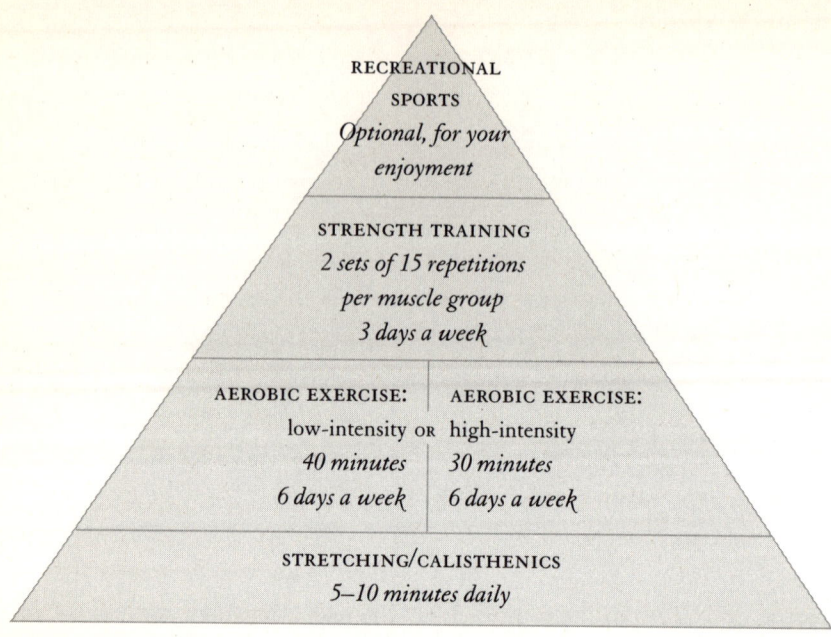

Figure 13.3 The Moderate-Risk Exercise Pyramid
The figure above illustrates the amounts of different types of exercise recommended for people in risk category level 3 (moderate risk).

LEVEL 4: HIGH RISK

You need to be still more aggressive and also more careful in your exercise program. On the aggressive side, you should increase your aerobic activity to a daily basis until your risk level has dropped. You should avoid competitive recreational sports. If you work diligently at the entire DEAR program, you will hopefully be able to resume these enjoyable sports activities soon. Remember to consult your health-care provider before starting any type of exercise and before resuming recreational sports.

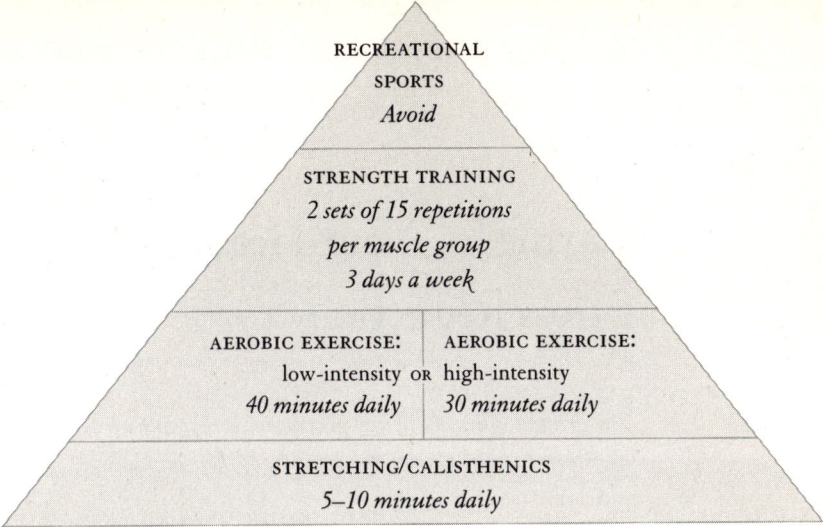

Figure 13.4 The High-Risk Exercise Pyramid
The figure above illustrates the amounts of different types of exercise recommended for people in risk category level 4 (high risk).

Putting It All Together

Exercise is an invaluable activity in its own right. However, when it comes to improving cardiovascular health, it works best as part of a total program. Exercise combined with a healthy diet is far more effective than either component alone. Chapter 16 will provide you with a series of worksheets you can use to record your activities and a stepwise program to increase your exercise to your target intensity and to the recommended amounts that best fit your profile.

 Caring for Your Heart: Stress Reduction

The greatest discovery of any generation is that human beings can alter their lives by altering the attitudes of their minds.
— ALBERT SCHWEITZER

Stress is known to be a major contributor to cardiovascular disease. In this chapter, we will look at ways to reduce your stress and give yourself the love, concern, and healing you deserve. Following the program outlined in this chapter will enhance your health and nurture you in all areas of your existence—physical, emotional, and spiritual. These are three components of a single being—you! You cannot experience feelings like anxiety, depression, guilt, or fear on a regular basis and expect to stay physically or spiritually healthy. You cannot assault your spirit without also affecting your physical and emotional well-being. And when your body is in a state of physical imbalance, you cannot expect your emotions and spirit to flourish. All three must work together and function well for you to be in optimum health. This chapter will explain what stress is, why it is detrimental to health, and how you can reduce the level of stress in your life and successfully manage those areas of stress that are unavoidable.

What Is Stress?

On the most basic level, existence and survival involve elements of stress. Walking, running, eating, breathing, making love, and indeed all activities put some degree of stress on the organs and systems involved. Of course, all of these activities are not unmitigated stressors. They are regenerating and healing, too. But because they cause changes in bodily functions and demand activity on the part of your organs and physical systems, they are stressful.

Scientists have discovered that even wonderful events, such as getting married, the arrival of a new baby, or a job promotion, can involve stress. Certainly the many day-to-day tasks that must be juggled can become very stressful. Balancing one's budget, dealing with teenage children, and getting to work on time are a few examples chosen at random from among the thousands of situations we confront every day. And, of course, major traumas such as divorce, the illness or death of a loved one, or sexual assault can be a dramatic source of enormous stress. An example of a major trauma we all shared is the events of September 11, 2001, which exacted a profound toll on the inner peace of many millions of people.

Ultimately, one cannot go through life without experiencing some stress. Defined simply, stress occurs when the body must leave its comfortable state of homeostasis and make some change. The greater the change, the more the stress. And the less desirable the change, the more damaging are the effects of that stress.

I say that the *body* makes a change, even when the stressor is a psychological event, such as the death of a loved one, because the mind, spirit, and body are closely linked. They cannot be separated into neat and discrete compartments. When you receive bad news or become angry, a series of physiological events is triggered.

The Effect of Stress on the Body

The process is an ancient one. It goes back to our prehistoric ancestors who lived in grassy plains and jungles. Like other creatures, they endured the minute-by-minute struggle for survival as they foraged for food, found or built shelters, and tried to keep safe from predators and natural disasters such as storms and floods. If one of our ancestors encountered a hungry lion, the body immediately snapped into action. Alerted to danger, the body primed itself to either fight the beast or flee from it. This is called the *fight-or-flight response.* The sympathetic nervous system goes on alert. The nerves and adrenal glands release two chemicals, called *epinephrine* and *norepinephrine,* which surge through the bloodstream raising blood pressure and increasing the heartbeat. Oxygen is delivered to the cells more rapidly and efficiently. Now the person is filled with energy and ready for intense physical activity.

This worked well in humanity's earliest environment, but it doesn't work so well in our so-called civilized society. We can't attack our teenage son when he misses his curfew and comes home with dents in the car (although perhaps we would like to). We can't run away from our glowering boss. But our heartbeat and physiology are screaming, "Fight, fight!" or "Run, run!" Our palms sweat, our heartbeat speeds up, we are breathless and raring to go.

This chain of events happens with varying degrees of intensity, depending on the nature of our emotional connection with the person or situation. If we have many stressors—work, home, schedule, or family—we may trigger the fight-or-flight response dozens of times daily. This takes a tremendous toll on cardiovascular health.

Getting an A in Stress

The stressors discussed above lie outside ourselves—a recalcitrant teenager, a nasty boss. But there are internal stressors, too. Some people react to innocuous situations by feeling threatened. The external structure of their lives is not dramatically stressful, but they are wired to spring into fight-or-flight mode at the slightest provocation, and even when there is no provocation. These individuals have what is known as a *type A personality*.

A is not a good grade to receive on your emotional report card. First identified by two cardiologists in the 1950s, the type A personality is chronically tense and anxious. Classically, type A people tend to be perfectionists about their work, punctuality, living space, and other situations. They react to life's day-to-day challenges by becoming angry or aggressive. Many studies have corroborated the impact that this pattern has on cardiovascular health.

Why is this so? Type A individuals experience the same ups and downs as the rest of us (a traffic jam, a bank error), but they interpret them in a manner that causes higher levels of stress. It's as if they are wearing distorted lenses. If you were wearing green eyeglasses, the world would appear green. Type A people see the world through glasses that make everything look menacing and problematic. A simple slip-up—for example, forgetting one's keys—becomes a major crisis. Type A personalities tend to drive themselves too hard and be perfectionistic. If they fall short, they blame themselves or someone else—or both.

The repeated bouts of anger and anxiety are extremely detrimental to the heart and blood vessels. The priming of the body for physical activity that never happens takes an enormous toll on the cardiovascular system. Interestingly, fats found in the bloodstream seem to rise and peak during times of stress. Studies of medical students, for example, reveal that they have the highest levels of serum fats during final examinations.

Receiving a D in Stress: Another Poor Grade

On the surface, depression might seem to be the opposite of stress. A depressed person is withdrawn and sad, while a type A person is anxious and irritable. However, depression has a negative effect on the body's chemistry and also places stress on the cardiovascular system. Individuals with depression are four times more likely than nondepressed people to develop CVD! There are many reasons for this, some indirect and others direct and causal.

Depression affects cardiovascular health in an indirect way because many depressed people engage in unhealthy behaviors such as overeating, smoking, and substance abuse. Depression also reduces motivation. If you are depressed, you are less likely to take good care of yourself. Exercise and healthy eating are often the first activities to be discarded.

Depression can be a personality style. Some people refer to it as the type D personality if a person is depressed because of turning anger against him- or herself. So if John's boss criticizes his report, John does not assert himself with his boss, or even allow himself to feel anger at being berated. Instead, he turns the anger on himself, believing that he is at fault. When his teenage daughter exceeds the limit on his credit card, John believes that he has been a bad parent; he must be if he has fathered such a disrespectful child. He is angry at himself rather than at his misbehaving child. This inverted anger—an emotion that should be directed at an outsider but instead is turned inward—translates into depression.

Depression can also be spawned by a sense of helplessness. John feels unable to change his work situation or assert himself with his daughter. He feels disempowered and out of control.

In John's case, depression is caused by his reaction to normal life circumstances. Depression is the gloom through which John sees the world. But depression can also be caused by external life circumstances. Social isolation is a great risk factor for developing depression and cardiovascular disease. So is CVD itself, and surgery (especially heart surgery). If you are recovering from a heart attack or bypass surgery, you are at risk for becoming depressed. It is a vicious cycle. Depressed people are more likely to have CVD, but CVD can induce depression. Whichever is the chicken and which the egg, one thing is clear: If you have had a heart attack or bypass surgery and you are depressed, your risk of having another heart attack—perhaps even a fatal one—rises by 50 percent.

Finally, certain medications can cause depression. What is especially disturbing is that some physicians fail to warn their patients of this side effect, believing that by providing this warning, they may plant ideas in the patient's head, as one doctor puts it. This is a grave disservice to patients who may suddenly feel sad without understanding why. Some blood pressure medications, for example, can have depression as a side effect. Many people erroneously believe that depression is a normal part of aging, or a normal reaction to illness or surgery. While it may be common, and in that sense normal, this does not mean it should be untreated!

Stress Reduction: A Synergistic Approach

Because stress is caused by external as well as internal factors, it must be addressed holistically and in multiple ways at once by adjusting both the external and the internal environment as much as possible. If your lifestyle is stressful, it will be harder for you to create and sustain a relaxed and peaceful inner state. Conversely, if you have a type A or type D personality, you will have a stressful inner state no matter what your external realities are. So it is important to tackle stress on all fronts simultaneously, making external changes and learning new ways to respond to situations that cannot be changed.

People have two physical legs on which they stand and walk; but it may surprise you to learn that we also have two emotional/spiritual "legs"—our stressors and our sources of resilience and strength. Learning to reduce your stress involves examining both legs, then strengthening the resiliency leg so that it does most of the walking.

Look at Your Stressors

Allow your mind to travel through the day-to-day realities of your life. And because it's easy to forget things, keep a log of your experiences. There are two ways to do this. Either take some quiet time to write down your activities, involvements, sources of pain and concern, and sources of pleasure and nurturance, or keep a running log as you go through your day. You may need to scribble things down or carry a tape recorder to speak into while you rush from one thing to the next. Your personality and lifestyle will determine which method works best for you. I encourage you to be creative and adapt this exercise to your own unique modes of expression.

As you do this, do not censor yourself. No stress is too minor or major to be included in your journal. The minor irritants can sometimes be as detrimental as the major problems if you allow them to get under your skin, and the cumulative effect of dealing with dozens of little nuisances can take a toll on your peace of mind.

At the end of this exercise, you should have a written account of your schedule, the people who populate your world, the thoughts and concerns that populate your mind and heart, and the issues that plague you on a regular basis. You should also have an indication of what resources—if any—you are using to give yourself strength, joy, and sustenance. For an example of what this might look like, see the Sample Daily Stress/Relaxation Log below.

Sample Daily Stress/Relaxation Log

It would not be possible to provide a single highly detailed set of guidelines for relaxation. Unlike food, supplements, and exercise, relaxation involves two components—attitude and actions. The attitude you take toward a situation will determine how stressful it is for you. For example, two people might both have an hour-long commute to work. One uses the time to relax by listening to enjoyable music or audiotapes, whether in the car or on the bus. A bus or train ride might be conducive to reading or meditation. Or perhaps he or she finds a travel companion and uses the time to socialize. Another person, however, might regard the commute as a stressor. Instead of using the time profitably, he or she fumes at traffic delays. Another example: Some people find dining alone after work to be a wonderful opportunity to unwind, while others who do so experience loneliness, boredom, or depression. The purpose of your stress/relaxation diary is to enable you to record *your* daily experiences, and the impact that they have on *you*. Following is a hypothetical diary.

BARBARA'S TUESDAY STRESS/RELAXATION LOG			
Time of Day	Activity	Feeling
6:00 A.M.	Alarm rings	Tired, angry, resentful. Went to bed too late, too many dishes, and the soccer uniform had to be washed for tonight's game. What got me up was reminding myself I could sleep on the bus on the way to work.
6:15 A.M.	Shower	The shower felt good. Nice hot water, lather.
6:45 A.M.	Wake kids	Annoyed and also happy. Joey got ready beautifully, but Tina took forever to get up, then she remembered she still had homework. I got mad. Yelled then felt terrible.
7:45 A.M.	Kids off to school, dishes	Angry about extra dishes but decided to wash them now instead of waiting until after work because of Joey's game—too much to do after work.
8:10 A.M.	Leave for work	Late because of taking extra time for dishes. Late to early meeting. Annie and Bruce mad at me.

This small diary segment shows a major stressor in Barbara's life. She is a single mother with two children, ages ten and fifteen. She cannot afford cleaning help and is overwhelmed by day-to-day tasks. After seeing how much stress the housework was causing her, she showed her children these pages of her diary, explaining that she needed their help and cooperation to reduce the stress in her life. For the first time,

(continued)

> the children felt like partners in a problem-solving process, rather than recipients of their mother's criticism. Barbara worked out a rotational system where she, Joey, and Tina took turns washing dishes. Barbara also realized how much she enjoyed her morning shower. Now that there were fewer dishes to wash, she was able to go to sleep earlier, wake up earlier, and take a longer shower. After discovering how good she felt during the shower, she purchased special soaps and shampoos to enhance her experience and when she stepped out of the shower in the mornings, she felt beautiful and invigorated. This is an example of how one woman's journal enabled her to identify a major daily stressor and an important source of relaxation, engage in some creative problem-solving, and reduce her stress while increasing the relaxation.

MAKE NECESSARY CHANGES

Now it's time to examine the stressors with an eye to making some changes. Is your schedule causing you daily stress? If so, how can it be altered? Perhaps this will involve tweaking or changing some other area of your life.

Some changes may be relatively simple, rather than dramatic and monumental. I know one man who was irritated every time he entered the kitchen because his wife had purchased a small wastepaper basket for kitchen use. The garbage was always overflowing and he was asked to empty it several times a day. He became annoyed every time he took out the trash. Buying a larger garbage can and presenting it to his wife made an enormous difference in his minute-to-minute peace of mind.

Some changes are harder to implement and require more creative thought. For example, if a coworker annoys you with endless chatter, perhaps you can request to be moved to a quieter office space. If you are under daily stress because you are saddled with too many household chores, perhaps you can ask your spouse and/or children to assume more of the respnsibility. If the morning commute causes you so much stress that you feel emotionally drained before you even set foot in the office, perhaps you should consider moving closer to work, asking for a transfer, or finding another job. If these are not options, perhaps you can alter your routine so that you get to bed earlier at night, wake up earlier in the morning, and beat the rush-hour madness. Sometimes getting up fifteen minutes earlier to beat the "bathroom rush" at home and taking a leisurely shower can make a great difference in the tone of your morning and of the entire day.

Of course, there are complex stressors that are difficult to address or alter because of potential financial, family, or other repercussions. An employment situation you hate, a cantankerous mother-in-law, and a child with a chronic illness are examples. I suggest that you use this as an opportunity to explore your beliefs about these situations and reduce the stress as much as possible. For example, I knew a family with an autistic child who needed constant supervision. The parents were exhausted. They decided to ask students from the special education department of the local college to help them so that they could get some respite. The students were happy to have experience in working with a special-needs child, and the parents had a reprieve from the unending demands of child care.

Although there are no hard-and-fast rules, your goal should be to have your perks outweigh your stressors, either qualitatively or quantitatively. To achieve this, you need to work on increasing your sources of resilience and relaxation as well as reducing your stress load. You can increase your relaxation by devoting more time to the things you enjoy, or by adding more things you enjoy to your day.

The parents in the earlier example used some of the time afforded by the presence of volunteer students to go to concerts and take nature walks, two important sources of pleasure and relaxation for them. It is important for you to identify *your* sources of strength and incorporate them into your life. Do you love to read? Sew? Do garden work? Do you have a hobby you're ignoring, such as stamp collecting or bird watching? It's time to attend to these neglected areas of pleasure and support. Sources of nurturance can be simple and don't have to be expensive—the hot drink while you do the crossword puzzle, a warm bath, taking a few minutes to talk to an old friend. If you are letting these things fall by the wayside in the daily hassle of your life, it is important to find ways of integrating them and increasing the time and focus you give them.

Making changes in your lifestyle—whether major or minor, whether these changes involve removing stressors or adding sources of pleasure—

often necessitates examining your assumptions. For example, the parents of the autistic child had always believed that caring for a child was a parent's job and should not be imposed on anyone else. They eventually concluded that there were others who could deliver excellent child care and that the time away from their child would enhance their physical and emotional health, their marriage, and their parenting. Staying in a job you hate because you think you cannot afford to leave may be objectively true, or it may be because you assume that you need a certain salary in order to sustain a set of "needs" that are really dispensable. Perhaps you will decide that it's more important to be in a pleasant and supportive work atmosphere, even if this involves a pay cut and a downscaled lifestyle for a while.

Some attitudinal work may turn some of your stresses into perks. For example, I know one woman who turned dishwashing into an enjoyable experience by bringing a boom box into the kitchen and listening to her favorite music while standing at the sink. The work sped by and she found she was actually disappointed when the sink was empty. This, in turn, led her to realize how important music was in her life and she began to consider returning to an old hobby, playing the piano, which she had left behind when she started college. If she decides to take up the piano again, she will be building something enjoyable and relaxing (a weekly music lesson) into her schedule, thereby adding yet another perk.

A WORD ABOUT SLEEP

It may emerge from your journal that you are not getting enough sleep. This is an aspect of self-care that deserves special mention, because the best program in the world will not work optimally if you are not sleeping enough. Your body needs sleep for the repair and regeneration of cells and tissues. Sleep enables all of your systems to function better, including your cardiovascular system. Lack of sleep has a directly damaging effect on the heart and blood vessels. In addition, when people don't sleep enough, they feel more stressed and irritable. They tend to make poorer decisions and have more trouble being creative in problem-solving. They also tend to drink more caffeinated beverages and to short-cut an energy rush by eating sugared foods. You know by now how detrimental these behaviors are to the heart.

How much sleep is enough? Again, there are no hard-and-fast rules, since we are all different, but sleep experts say that most people need between six and eight hours per night. If your schedule cannot accommodate this, you may be able to make up for lost sleep by taking regular naps at the same time each day.

Counseling: Helping to Change Externals, Helping to Change Internals

The journaling and reflection exercise outlined above is only a beginning. You may find yourself facing major issues, even in relatively minor areas. For example, if the man who replaced the kitchen garbage was afraid that his wife would have a tantrum because he was defying her and therefore chose to "put up and shut up," he would need to address the fundamental issues in his marriage. Certainly, major life changes such as leaving a job, ending a marriage, or arranging for an elderly relative to live in a nursing home can involve many complex beliefs about yourself, your obligations and commitments, and the world in which you live. You may not be able to do this without extra support and assistance—which brings us to the subject of counseling.

Some people, especially older adults, still believe that counseling and psychotherapy are for "crazy people." Others feel that counseling is simply useless and won't address the problems in their lives. They say, "No headshrinker can change what's bothering me [my no-good son, my rotten boss], so why bother with counseling?"

Nothing could be further from the truth. In fact, it requires emotional maturity to reach out for help. Doing so is a sign of health and sanity, not craziness. And talking about a problem can often bring relief even if there is no immediate solution in sight. Often, sharing an apparently insoluble situation with an objective and experienced professional can help you gain new perspective and see options that had not occurred to you before. You may then be able to take steps that you never thought possible.

Counseling can also help you to change deep-seated personality styles that are impeding your functioning. If you are a type A or type D person, you can alter these destructive ways of taking in the world.

There are many different types of counseling. The stereotypical "shrink" to which many of my older patients refer derives from the early Freudian psychoanalytic model, in which the patient lies on the couch, free-associating about early toilet training, while a silent and morose analyst sits behind the couch taking notes. I am not denigrating the value of psychoanalysis, but there are many other forms of therapy that are more focused, accomplish their goals more rapidly, and are more interactive. These include psychodynamic psychotherapy and cognitive behavioral therapy.

Many different types of professionals are qualified to offer counseling, including psychiatrists, psychologists, social workers, certified counselors, and members of the clergy. Depending on your needs, you might also consider a marriage counselor or a support group. For example, if you are dealing with a relative who suffers from Alzheimer's disease, a group for caregivers might give you emotional support and practical guidance. The Resources section will give you tips for finding a counselor who meets your needs.

Nonverbal Therapeutic Approaches

Talk therapy isn't for everyone. Some people simply are not verbal communicators. They do not find talking about problems to be helpful. These people are often criticized by others for not sharing their feelings. This places additional pressure on them, which compounds whatever problems they are already dealing with. There are some excellent therapeutic approaches that do not rely on verbal communication as the primary mechanism for effecting change. Following are a few examples.

ART THERAPY, DANCE/MOVEMENT THERAPY, AND MUSIC THERAPY

These approaches use the artistic media of art, dance and physical movement, or music to express and process feelings, release traumas, and tap into personal creativity. You do not need to be a professional artist, dancer, or musician to benefit. The goal is expression, not performance. Of course, if your hobby or profession is music, dance, or art, so much the better.

EYE MOVEMENT DESENSITIZATION AND REPROCESSING

Eye movement desensitization and reprocessing (EMDR) uses a series of eye movements to replicate the neurological state of rapid eye movement (REM) sleep while addressing a problem or trauma. Francine Shapiro, Ph.D., psychologist and creator of this approach, discovered that if one duplicated the eye movements characteristic of this phase of sleep while focusing on a negative image, distressing thought, or unpleasant sensation, the negative impact of the event lessened and the individual found different ways of processing the experience. In practice, this involves holding in mind a representative image of a problem while watching the practitioner's hand or a light that moves in a rhythmic manner. Individuals who have not found talk-based approaches helpful have reported experiencing relief from stress and enhanced problem-solving abilities after treatment with EMDR. This approach has been gaining credibility in scientific circles.

SOMATIC EXPERIENCING

This is a modality created by psychologist Peter A. Levine, Ph.D. It takes a body-based approach to stress and trauma. According to Dr. Levine, trauma imprints itself upon the survivor's physiology, not only his or her psyche. This is especially the case if the fight-or-flight response to trauma is aborted because the person could neither fight nor escape the threatening situation. The uncompleted movement must be released for healing to occur. In somatic experiencing, you are taught how to focus on your bodily sensations and to discharge "frozen" movement patterns. Please note that any event that the individual perceives as a threat is regarded as traumatic; the term is not limited to the type of dramatic, life-threatening events we typically associate with the word *trauma*.

Relaxation Techniques

Sources of stress cannot always be eliminated. If you have examined your lifestyle and concluded that there are stressors you cannot avoid, the next step is to find ways of reducing the damaging effects that these stressors have on your system. And because you're human, you will discover that it is impossible to live a completely stress-free life. This is why it is so important to learn relaxation techniques. Which one or ones you choose will depend on your lifestyle, as well as your personal orientation and spiritual outlook, because many of these techniques have been derived from ancient spiritual traditions. Ultimately, the purpose of all these techniques is to create what Harvard Medical School cardiologist Herbert Benson, M.D., called the *relaxation response*. When you are relaxed, it actually changes your body chemistry, which has far-reaching implications for your whole body, especially your cardiovascular system.

On a biochemical level, when you relax, your brain shifts into a different mode of action. The brain waves that are produced when you are relaxed are different from those produced when you are asleep, working, running around, or feeling anxious. Neurologists have identified four different types of brain waves, which are designated alpha, beta, gamma, and theta waves. The brain produces alpha waves during periods of deep relaxation.

When the brain is in an alpha state, the entire body shifts as well. The body's metabolic rate decreases and less oxygen is needed and consumed. The heartbeat slows down. The blood vessels dilate, which is especially beneficial to those with high blood pressure. This happens during sleep as well, but during sleep, the brain is producing several different types of waves at different stages of sleep. Each stage produces a different metabolic rate, and none of the sleep waves is as profoundly restful to the body as the alpha waves produced during deep relaxation. So although sleep is important for the regeneration of many bodily systems, including the cardiovascular system, it is not a substitute for relaxation.

As mentioned earlier, many relaxation techniques derive from ancient spiritual practices. Indeed, some of the pioneering research on the relaxation response was conducted by studying practitioners of yoga, which is derived from the Hindu tradition. There are, however, techniques and approaches that have sought to secularize religious practices. You can use whichever type of technique is most consistent with your own philosophy.

BIOFEEDBACK

Biofeedback uses sensitive machinery to show which type of waves your brain is producing. Sensors attached to your head record brain waves and translate them into an image on a monitor or screen. This image gives you feedback about what is happening in your body. Your goal is to get the image on the screen to confirm that you are producing alpha waves and to learn how to produce these waves at will. While biofeedback is usually conducted in an office setting, with the assistance of a trained specialist, you can try it on your own as well. Small hand-held monitors are available for home use. Ideally, the skill of inducing deep relaxation becomes transferable to other situations, even when no biofeedback equipment is available. So during stressful moments, you can generate the relaxation response to counterbalance your body's instinctive fight-or-flight response.

MEDITATION

Meditation is a powerful and versatile tool. Unlike biofeedback, you don't need any special equipment to do it. Meditation is a great way to start your day if you are an early riser, or a great way to finish the day if you function better at night. If you experience stress during the day, meditation can be a wonderful way to calm yourself. Although it is best to meditate for at least twenty minutes at a stretch, even shorter periods will be helpful if that's not possible.

There are many different forms of meditation. The purpose of all methods is to calm the mind and its endless chatter so as to allow the profound state of relaxation, with its alpha waves, to prevail. Although meditation was traditionally performed in a cross-legged position, it's fine to sit in a straight-backed chair as well. Lying down is fine except that it makes it easier to fall asleep. And although it has its roots in Eastern religious traditions, scientists such as Dr. Benson have Westernized and secularized it. He adapted a technique called Transcendental Meditation (TM), which involves repeating and concentrating on a sound or a word (traditionally called a *mantra*) again and again. In TM, the mantra is assigned to the meditator by a teacher, but Dr. Benson encouraged people to select any word or sound that is meaningful to them.

Alternative meditational approaches designed to accomplish the same goal involve concentrating one's attention on an object (such as a flower, candle, picture, or holy item), listening to soothing sounds (such as gentle music or natural settings—you can obtain recorded ocean waves, for example), or concentrating on your breathing. An easy Zen technique involves counting your breaths, beginning with 1 and going to 10. If you become distracted, you begin again. At first, you may not get beyond the number 2. But as you practice, your concentration will deepen, and eventually you will find yourself counting all the way. Additional resources can be found on page 291.

EXERCISE-BASED MEDITATION

On the surface, it would appear that exercise and meditation are contradictions, since one involves activity and one is designed to produce a calm state of mind through inactivity. But this is not accurate. There are ancient meditational approaches that enhance concentration and create the relaxation response through using various body motions and exercises. These include tai chi and qigong, two practices that originated in China, and yoga, which originated in India. Most of the martial arts, such as judo, jujitsu, tae kwon do, aikido, and kung fu also contain meditational components. Finally, you can do walking meditation. This differs from power walking, which is designed to stimulate your heart to beat faster and your body to use oxygen more efficiently. This is a gentle, slow process called *kin hin* in Zen tradition.

THE ROLE OF LAUGHTER

In his book *Anatomy of an Illness as Perceived by the Patient* (W.W. Norton, 2001), Norman Cousins described his battle with a serious disease called ankylosing spondylitis. One of the most important tools he used was laughter. He watched comedies and attributed much of the success in overcoming his illness to the role of laughter. Patch Adams, author of *Gesundheit!* (Inner Traditions International, 1998), is a doctor who used humor extensively in his work with patients. Robin Williams starred in a movie about his life and the positive impact his sense of humor had on his patients.

Scientists have actually researched why laughter has such a profound impact on the system. For example, a group of students at a Malaysian university participated in a nine-day study of laughter therapy. At the end of this time, they reported improved appetite, greater relaxation, and better sleep patterns. They also reported greater self-confidence during final examinations.

I urge you to find contexts in which to laugh. This does not mean ignoring areas of pain or struggle, of course. Bernie Siegel, M.D., best-selling author of *Love, Medicine and Miracles* (Perennial Press, 1998), distinguishes between using laughter as therapy and using laughter as an escape from all problems, pain, or unresolved issues. But going to see a comedy, renting funny videos, reading joke books, or just having fun is wonderful therapy. So don't feel guilty about taking time from your busy day to relax and have a good time. It's doctor's orders!

BODY-BASED RELAXATION TECHNIQUES

Although we generally regard stress as a mental state, we know that its effects live in the body because, as we have seen throughout this chapter, the mind and body are not two disconnected entities but are part of the same larger entity—you. Emotional disturbances can lodge themselves in the body and manifest themselves as physical problems, including cardiovascular problems. Often, by working directly with the body, the negative effects of stress can be reversed. Bodywork can even help you deal more effectively with stresses in the future and not become so stressed-out by challenging situations. Following are brief summaries of some different types of body-based approaches.

Acupuncture and Shiatsu

Acupuncture originated in China nearly five thousand years ago. It involves the use of hair-fine needles applied to specific points of the body to help revitalize or unblock the life force or energy flow, which the Chinese refer to as *qi*. Acupuncture is rapidly becoming more popular in the United States and elsewhere in the world as well. It has been particularly useful in treating chronic pain and can help reduce the necessity for medications. There are acupuncture techniques that specifically address tension and can help induce deep relaxation. If you are squeamish or uncomfortable about the needles used in traditional acupuncture, there is an alternative. You might find that a form of acupressure known as *shiatsu* is more suitable. Shiatsu involves the application of finger pressure to specific points on the body in a firm, rhythmic sequence to awaken acupuncture meridians.

Massage

Massage involves pressing, stroking, or manipulating your muscles and skin to improve the flow of energy, blood, and lymph. Massage feels wonderful. It can be very relaxing, soothing, stress-reducing, and pain-relieving. It can help improve your circulation, immune response, headaches, injuries, and other difficulties.

Bodywork

There are a variety of different techniques that come under the umbrella of the term *bodywork*. They are all designed to improve your flexibility, increase your range of motion, and allow your body to move easily and freely. Bodywork techniques require hands-on manipulation by a skilled practitioner. Some of these include Rolfing, the Alexander Technique, and the Feldenkrais Method. On the other hand, techniques involving energy medicine may not require hands-on treatment and may not involve any touching at all. This form of healing is still very controversial. Energy methods are thought to release blocked energy and to restore normal body functioning.

Connection with Others

The incidence of mortality from cardiovascular disease is dramatically higher than average in isolated individuals. People fare better in communities than in isolation. Throughout history, people were usually interconnected. People lived in tribal groups, close-knit communities, and/or extended families. Joys, sorrows, and practical chores such as farming, laundering, hunting, and child care were shared. Elders were not discarded but were venerated, and young children were cared for by everyone. ("It takes a village...") If we look at many non-Western countries, we see that this lifestyle has been continued among indigenous populations. In Western societies, however, the legacy of the Puritan concept of rugged individualism is that many of us become isolated. We have the technology to live alone, and our society places a great emphasis on autonomy and independence. The result is that many of us are lonely and disconnected from others, especially as we grow older.

If you live alone, this is a good time to reach out to others. If you don't drive, you can probably arrange alternate forms of transportation. Most cities have some type of transportation services for seniors, and even those that don't usually have churches or civic groups that may be willing to step in and provide wheels. There are many wonderful ways to meet new people and make friends, whatever your age. If you are trying to incorporate aerobic exercise into your life, consider joining a gym or walking group. If you have a hobby such as sewing or reading, consider joining a club. If you are a senior, you might look into events at local community or senior centers. If you are religiously oriented, consider joining a church, synagogue, or other house of worship and becoming involved in their programs. And whatever your background, age, or interests, you can always find a way to volunteer. Volunteering gives you a sense of meaning and also serves as a social setting for developing new friendships.

As with removing lifestyle stressors, which would involve creative thinking and challenge entrenched beliefs and assumptions, if you have led an isolated life for a long time, it may be difficult for you to make changes. You may feel shy and awkward starting conversations with new people, or reluctant to impose upon others by asking them to drive you to your destinations. I urge you to overcome these feelings of anxiety and explore new aspects of yourself. You have a lot to gain from developing friendships—and your newfound friends will gain a great deal from you as well.

THE ROLE OF SPIRITUALITY

One of the most striking responses to the events of September 11, 2001, was how many Americans turned to religion for solace. Churches were filled to overflowing during the weeks and months following the attack, and spiritual counselors were greatly sought after by families of the victims, as well as by members of the general population. Numerous studies support the fact that belonging to a religious structure of some sort and having a strong faith confer measurable health benefits. Other studies point to the positive effects that prayer has on heartbeat, relaxation, and respiration. Ultimately, prayer and other spiritual activities can help you feel connected to a force greater than yourself. This connection is a source of support and comfort and has measurable and demonstrable health benefits.

Even if you don't believe in a specific religion, it is important to nurture your spirit in ways that feel meaningful to you. For example, natural beauty, poetry, and music are examples of things that most people find inspiring. In addition, having an organizing principle in life helps create a sense of well-being and meaning that goes beyond the daily stressors. Psychiatrist and Holocaust survivor Viktor Frankl wrote that those who had a sense of purpose withstood the horrors of the concentration camp far better than those who did not. Find a greater purpose or an activity that moves you and brings you meaning and comfort, and you will be taking care of your spirit as well as your heart.

At the root of all great spiritual traditions is a vision of unconditional love. Whatever context you choose, if you tap into that vision and extend this blessing to everyone in your life, you will experience greater healing and inner peace. Don't forget to include yourself, of course! The more you find ways to love yourself and others, the more connected you will be with the source of all spirituality. Creating a relaxed environment is a product of creating a synergistic and harmonious relationship between mind, body, and spirit. Putting these suggestions to work in your life can literally help to heal your broken heart.

 15   Obstacles to Self-Care

Ride on over all obstacles and win the race!
—Charles Dickens

Most of my patients come to me knowing that it's bad for them to eat a high-fat diet or to be overweight. They have learned this from the media and from their doctors. I hear groans when they tell me, "I know I *should* be cutting down on fat," or, "The last doctor I saw already told me I need to lose weight." These people come to see me because, ostensibly, they would like to be healthier. But something prevents them from turning their desire for good health into a committed and consistent lifestyle. In this chapter we will look at some of the most common obstacles that get in the way of translating good intentions into practice.

Lack of Motivation

Jed, age forty-two, consulted me because he was concerned about his elevated cholesterol and triglycerides and strong family history of heart disease. Jed's father had died of a heart attack at age forty-five. His uncle had died of heart disease at age forty-seven and his grandfather at fifty. At five feet, four inches and 193 pounds, Jed was overweight. His doctor prescribed atorvastatin (Lipitor), but Jed stopped taking it because he was experiencing muscle aches and fatigue, and blood tests showed elevated liver enzymes. Jed was worried about discontinuing the medication because of his high risk for heart disease. He seemed eager to find alternatives to statin drugs for cholesterol reduction.

I introduced Jed to the DEAR program and gave him a series of guidelines for implementing and personalizing the program to suit his high-risk profile. We wrote out a diet and I sent him home with a suggested meal plan. We agreed that he would start a walking regimen— four days a week for twenty minutes. I gave him a list of supplements with instructions regarding dosage, and I urged him to make more time for recreation.

At his next appointment, Jed's lab test results were disturbing. His total cholesterol had risen from 240 to 304 and his triglycerides from 409 to 652. He had put on six pounds. "What happened?" I asked in dismay.

"I don't have time for all these changes," he said defensively. "Who can eat brown rice and sprouts? You need a knife and fork and you can't use the computer at the same time. A sandwich works better. And I'm much too busy to exercise." Still, he promised to try to do better.

At his next visit, three months later, he reported that he had significantly improved his diet and started using some of the supplements I had recommended, although he still was not exercising. His blood test results showed some mild improvement. But his numbers were still far too high, so I encouraged him to begin exercise and relaxation regimens and try harder to follow his diet.

The next appointment, a year later, was initiated by Jed's wife, who accompanied him to my office. Jed had gained weight, his cholesterol and triglycerides were dramatically elevated, and hs-CRP was a staggering 4.44. Jed explained this by saying he had gotten transferred to another department at work with even more pressure, so he had no time to exercise, practice relaxation, or eat properly.

"Why do you work so hard?" I asked Jed.

He looked surprised. "What kind of question is that? Why does anyone work? To put food on the table. So my family can have a good life. So my kids can go to college."

"If you don't change your lifestyle, you may not live to see your kids graduate from college," I said. I didn't like being so blunt, but with Jed, I felt I had no choice.

Jed was visibly shaken. After this visit, he began taking the dietary program more seriously and noticed rapid results in a matter of weeks. He felt more energetic and lost over thirty pounds. Plus, his levels of cholesterol, triglycerides, and hs-CRP all dropped—not yet to the healthiest range, but there was a significant improvement. Then he began to exercise and took his supplements religiously. He also became committed to incorporating more relaxation into his life. To do this, he knew that his work situation would have to change. He went to see his supervisor, asking for a more humane schedule. She refused, so he requested and received a transfer to a lower-pressure department. To his surprise, he found that his wife and children were so happy to see more of him that they didn't mind doing without some of the luxuries they were used to, and his marriage and sex life improved. And ultimately, his blood test results all came down to within the normal range.

Jed's story illustrates the first obstacle in implementing my program: lack of motivation. He had become a workaholic in order to meet his mental image of being a good father and provider. But his real organizing principle was love for his children and commitment to their well-being. Once he realized that his lifestyle could damage them instead of helping them, he finally had the motivation to make the necessary changes.

"But There's No Time!"

I can't tell you how often I've heard this reason—or excuse—for not adhering to the DEAR program. Most of my patients lead high-stress lives, and time is their most precious commodity. They say there is no time to cook properly, exercise, or engage in relaxation. But in my experience, this is simply a variant of low motivation.

Kristine, age thirty-nine, is a good example of someone who came to see me because her cholesterol and triglycerides were too high (262 and 178, respectively). Although she did not have any symptoms of CVD, her primary care physician was worried about the family history; Kristine's mother had died at the age of thirty-six of Wolff-Parkinson-White disease, a form of cardiac disease. Her father suffered from hypertension and had recently sustained a series of disabling strokes. "The doctor wants me to take medication, but I've read some bad things about that stuff, so I came here," she said.

When I outlined my program to her, she shook her head. "I can't do that," she said. "Between my job and the kids and my father, I have no time for myself." She outlined a frenetic schedule that involved juggling the complicated needs of her work and her responsibilities as a divorced mother to three children and daugher of an aging and ailing father.

I decided to explore the "no time for myself" issue with her. No matter what practical suggestion I made, it was met with a series of reasons why this was unworkable. Most of these arguments centered around the inability of anyone but her to care for her children or father. At last I asked her why she believed she was the only one who could provide adequate care to these family members.

Kristine burst into tears. She admitted that she felt guilty about her mother's death—she had been at the movies when it happened—and had convinced herself that she needed to be more present for her family. I advised her to get counseling around her guilt and explore how it was impeding her ability to take care of her own health now.

At Kristine's next appointment, five months later, her total cholesterol and triglycerides had both come down. They were not yet ideal, but she was committed to working on her health. She was sharing childcare responsibilities more equally with her ex-husband, and several volunteers from the community checked up on her father when she was at the gym.

Like Jed, Kristine was an example of an individual who claimed to have no time to take care of her health, but who was really impeded by some other underlying belief about time management and self-care. We all go through periods of crisis in our lives when there really is no time for exercise or healthy cooking, but when people lead *consistently* high-stress, low-time lifestyles, something else is almost always going on.

"But I Don't Have Any Willpower!"

Lack of willpower, like a lack of time, is an excuse people use when they are unwilling to face some other issue or belief. Although it is ostensibly a statement that implies assuming responsibility for weakness, it is actually a subtle attempt to shift blame onto the missing ingredient—willpower. Investigating what lies beneath the lack of this elusive thing called willpower often yields important results. Why is eating tasty food more important than a commitment to good health or an attractive appearance? Maybe because good health or attractiveness is threatening for some reason. Some people are afraid of being attractive, for example, because of unresolved sexual or emotional issues. Some people are afraid of feeling too healthy or successful. Perhaps illness or weakness has given them the attention they lack or the nurturing they otherwise could not receive.

A similar phenomenon often happens with older people, who frequently have a push-pull relationship with dependence. On the one hand, they do not want to be a burden to family members, but on the other hand, they may be comfortable with the dependent role and fear that if they are too independent, their needs may not be met.

Dorothea was a fifty-eight-year-old woman who had diabetes. Her religious training led her to believe that it was her responsibility to take care of her family's household needs. She had always catered to her husband and her children and put her own needs second. Even once her children were independent adults, she continued to wait on her husband hand and foot. Only when she was ill could she enjoy a reprieve from her enormous list of responsibilities. Dorothea completely refused to follow my program, claiming that she had no willpower. I knew of her Herculean schedule and believed that that was what underlay her apparent lack of willpower. When her triglycerides reached an astounding 1,050 (one of the highest levels I had ever encountered), I recommended family therapy with a clergy member.

Dorothea may be an extreme example, but in my experience most people who claim to lack willpower really lack a commitment to good health. They harbor a fear or a self-defeating belief of which they are not aware. Only by uncovering what is really going on can you build your willpower and adhere to a lifestyle that is in your best interest. Lack of willpower does not manifest itself only when it comes to dieting. It requires willpower to sustain a regular exercise regimen, for example. "I'm lazy," one of my patients said frankly. Often, as in the case of Dorothea, there are deep-seated psychological reasons for this.

"I Just Can't Give Up My Favorite Foods"

Of the four components of my program, the one most consistently difficult for people to follow is diet. Although it is challenging to incorporate exercise and relaxation into your life, it is still easier than altering long-standing eating habits. My patients consistently report feeling a sense of deprivation, especially when they must give up their favorite foods. Here are some of the issues that they raise:

COMFORT

From earliest childhood, we learn to associate certain foods with emotional comfort. Perhaps we remember Mom holding out a steaming cup of hot chocolate or Dad buying us a hot dog at a ballgame. When we are upset as adults, we reflexively turn to those foods that evoke these warm, happy associations as a way of giving ourselves love.

The key to overcoming this obstacle is to realize that by giving yourself unhealthy comfort foods you are not really showing love for yourself. You must recognize that there are many ways to show self-love and you must learn new ways to find comfort—say, taking a walk in the park, taking a bath, reading a book, listening to music, or whatever. One of my friends who has had a lifelong weight problem has learned to manage it by wearing soft, cozy clothing. Or perhaps you can reach for the phone and call a friend if you are upset, instead of reaching for the refrigerator door.

Bertha, age forty-eight, was seventy-five pounds overweight and had been on a diet all her adult life, but had never managed to lose the weight. Every time she got upset, she said, she found herself at the table, sitting over a dish of butter pecan ice cream without even remembering how it got there. I told her to slow things down and watch the process unfold. It turned out that when she was upset, she automatically turned to a food she had enjoyed as a child. She learned to catch herself when the distressed feelings first set in and to substitute other activities.

It requires some relearning and rewiring of our accustomed associations to make these changes. Make a list of your favorite activities and your favorite things. Create a plan so that when you are upset, you have an armamentarium of substitutes for eating the things you shouldn't. This can include nibbling on healthy foods, as well as activities or objects that give you pleasure.

INDEPENDENCE AND AUTONOMY

Many of us have evolved a lifestyle with which we are pleased and proud. We associate this lifestyle with making it in life. We are driving the car we always wanted to drive, we are living in the neighborhood we always dreamed of, we can eat whatever we want to and refuse whatever we don't like. We don't have to eat our spinach any more because we are adults now. One patient of mine refused to exercise because he was forced to walk everywhere when he was a child. Another exulted in pulling out the soft insides of bread because she was never allowed to do this as a child.

Ellen, thirty-four, was thirty pounds overweight, tired, and depressed. Although her cholesterol was normal, her triglyceride levels were extremely high—in the 900s. She also had elevated homocysteine levels. Diabetes and cardiovascular disease ran in her family, but she refused to change her diet.

I could not understand her stubbornness, given her high level of risk, until she explained that when she was a child, her parents doled out her food and there was no arguing. She was not allowed to help herself to food, nor was she allowed to refuse it. "I'm never going to let anyone tell me what to eat again," she told me.

Some of my patients have lived through the Depression or suffered from poverty or food rationing for other reasons. To voluntarily deprive themselves of favorite foods in times of prosperity makes no sense to them. Complex emotional issues like these (and Ellen's) often require counseling.

HABIT

Many of us have developed a series of habits that are, for the most part, quite good for us. We don't have to walk ourselves through the activities of brushing our teeth or turning the ignition key in the car. These are things we do automatically. Eating certain foods often falls into the same category. Many of us pour the cornflakes into our bowl, the milk onto the cornflakes, and the sugar on top of both without much thought, while we read the morning paper. Food is one of the things we'd rather *not* think about.

I have found guidance in handling this area from meditational approaches, such as those of mindfulness meditation. These stress the importance of awareness of each moment as an opportunity for self-love and connection with ourselves and others. Instead of mindlessly rushing through routinized activities, we slow down and focus on them. It is amazing how much more pleasure you will get out of your food if you take a few minutes to eat slowly, chew your food thoroughly, and focus on the flavor and texture of each bite. People have told me that when they really stop to enjoy the foods they eat, they feel more satisfied. They also feel less need for foods that are bad for their health and find more pleasure in foods that nurture their health.

"IT'S WEIRD"

As Americans, we are accustomed to certain foods that are part of our society. Learning new eating patterns feels strange at first. Some people associate a diet that is high in vegetables, whole grains, and plant- or fish-based protein with "weird," "alternative," or "New Age" lifestyles and shy away from the connotations of this type of diet.

Although many people involved in so-called alternative lifestyles are also more health-conscious than many other Americans, there is no logical association between any particular political or philosophical orientation and eating a healthy diet. It helps to remember that throughout the centuries, these healthier foods were the predominant—in fact the only—foods that most people ate. It is only in the last one hundred years or so that increasingly processed foods have made their way into the marketplace, and only in the last hundred years that cardiovascular disease has become so prevalent.

Likewise, there is nothing inherently manly about the typical American diet. I'm always disturbed when a patient refers to himself as a "meat-and-potatoes man," as if eating tofu or salad casts aspersions on his masculinity. You will not feel very manly if you are fatigued or laid up in the hospital after a heart attack. The healthier you are, the more vigorous, energetic, and powerful you will feel.

FOOD CRAVINGS

Sometimes, we have urges to eat particular foods. Although there can be psychological reasons for these, there can also be physiological reasons, such as nutritional or metabolic imbalances. For example, one of my patients was a "cheesaholic." Amy was addicted to hard cheese in any form. She also enjoyed other forms of fatty foods. You can imagine what that did to her cholesterol levels. I theorized that perhaps she was not metabolizing her fats correctly and therefore craved fatty foods. Remember, the body needs a certain amount of fat to carry out basic functions. My guess was that while she was eating large quantities of fat, she was not absorbing them. So I recommended L-carnitine supplements, together with digestive enzymes designed to break down dietary fat. I also asked her to reduce her consumption of saturated fats and increase her intake of the omega-3 fatty acids, both in supplements and in foods. Amy was subsequently amazed the first time she took her children out to pizza and was able to resist the temptation.

If you persistently crave a particular type of food, it is worth discussing this with your health-care provider or nutritionist. There may be a metabolic component, such as food allergies or malabsorption, that can be addressed.

Additional Approaches to Overcoming Obstacles

Acupuncture is extremely helpful for many eating issues. There are specific types of acupuncture designed to address addictions, including food addictions. Others address food cravings, and others can help achieve feelings of peace and tranquility. Guided imagery and hypnosis can help you behaviorally and can also help you uncover the reasons you overeat. You can see a professional hypnotist, attend a class, or purchase tapes or books.

Fill out the worksheets in chapter 16 to gain a clearer idea of the obstacles that may be stopping you from adhering to a program that could both save your life and improve your quality of life. Ultimately, I think it boils down to a decision to retrain yourself so that you see this program as the best way of giving yourself love. Then you will have already won half the battle.

 16   DEAR Diary: Your Personal Workbook

Look in thy heart and write.
—Sir Philip Sidney

This chapter is designed to help you put your complete program together. It is your personal workbook for implementing the things you have learned in the previous chapters. As you become more comfortable with your new lifestyle, you may not need to journal your foods and activities every day, because they will become second nature to you.

Before beginning this process, refer back to the risk-factor questionnaire you filled out in chapter 9, if necessary, and record your point score and risk category here:

- My risk factor point score (fill in): _____
- My risk category (check one):
    _____ 1: Prevention   _____ 2: Low Risk
    _____ 3: Moderate Risk   _____ 4: High Risk

The pages that follow contain blank templates of journals for you to fill in. I encourage you to leave the pages in the book blank and make photocopies for your personal journal. You can keep them in a folder or use a three-hole punch and store your pages in a binder.

Diet Diaries

There are two different formats here for keeping your diet record. One is the standard daily food log similar to those you will find in most diet books and nutritionists' offices. The other is a daily food pyramid, with a weekly and monthly side comment section for those foods you cannot have on a daily basis, but are allowed on a weekly or monthly basis.

Why two formats? Because I have learned from colleagues who are nutritionists and dietitians, and from my own clinical experience, that people easily forget what they have eaten in the course of a day. The nibbled cookie, the second helping of meatloaf, the extra-large serving of fries . . . it's easy to lose track of what we eat. Seeing it in black and white on paper helps us to remember. Additionally, a written food journal helps you organize your daily menus and food plans.

The pyramid helps you see if you are getting enough servings on a daily basis of the various categories and food groups that will advance your therapeutic program. Coordinating the two diaries will enable you to construct a food lifestyle for yourself.

As your health improves, your risk category will, hopefully, change. When it does, you can put aside your higher-risk food pyramids and begin using lower-risk templates. But don't throw away your earlier diaries. They will give you a basis of comparison as you move through your health plan. Then, if you should start to feel discouraged or deprived, you can look back and see how far you have come. Additionally, if you encounter an unexpected health snag or problem that places you in a higher-risk group, you have earlier menus to refer to.

Daily Food Diary

WEEK STARTING: _____ ENDING: _____

RISK LEVEL: ____	MONDAY	TUESDAY	WEDNESDAY	THURSDAY	FRIDAY	SATURDAY	SUNDAY
BREAKFAST							
MIDMORNING SNACK							
LUNCH							
AFTERNOON SNACK							
DINNER							
DESSERT OR EVENING SNACK							

Exercise Diaries

Your exercise diary, like your food diary, has two components: a daily journal to help you chart the amount and type of exercise you are doing on a daily basis, and a weekly pyramid to help you organize and keep track of your exercise program. Again, make photocopies of the blank template pages and use them to create your own personal exercise record, writing down the type of exercise and the amount of time spent on each exercise.

Nutritional Supplementation Diary

This section is constructed a little differently from the sections on diet and exercise. Although there are pyramids for the categories of diet and exercise, I find that the most useful way to organize a supplement regimen is through a log that covers the supplements of a single day. Here you will find a blank log page for each risk level, listing the supplements recommended for each. Make photocopies of the appropriate page to create your personal supplementation diary. Refer to chapter 12 for appropriate dosage levels.

A few caveats: Remember that you should start by taking the lowest recommended dosage of each supplement and then gradually increase the dosage if necessary. Remember, too, that not everyone will need all of the supplements listed for that risk level. This is particularly true for people in the moderate-risk and high-risk categories, where some of the supplements address specific risk factors and symptoms. Again, refer to chapter 12 to see if your symptoms necessitate the use of any given supplement. Finally, as you move through the program, you will, hopefully, require fewer supplements and lower dosages of the supplements you are continuing to take. When that happens, adjust your journal accordingly.

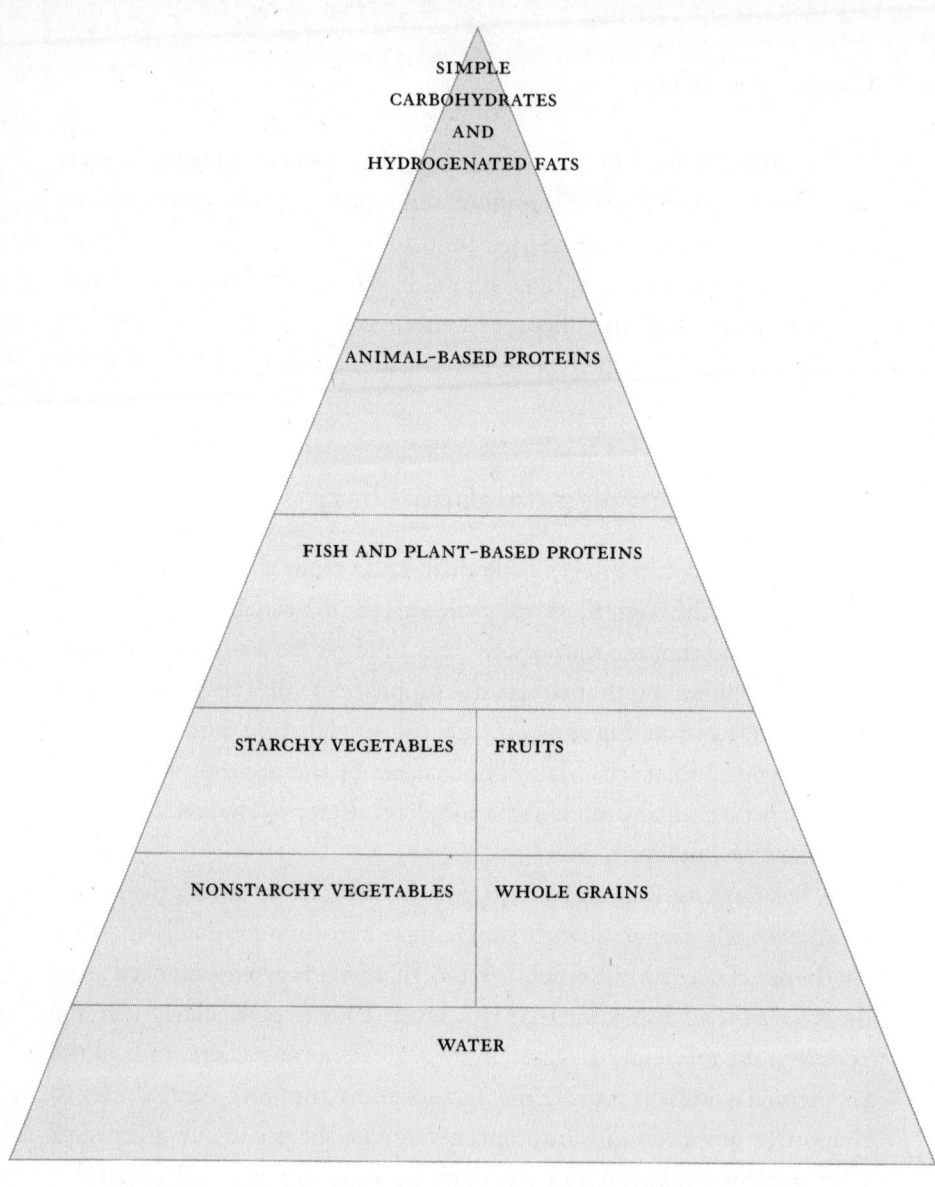

Food Diary Pyramid

Make photocopies of this page and use it to record your daily servings of foods in each of the pyramid categories (refer back to the appropriate food pyramid in chapter 11 to remind yourself of the appropriate number of servings of each for your risk level). You can also use the blank pyramid to help you create menu plans that fulfill your dietary goals.

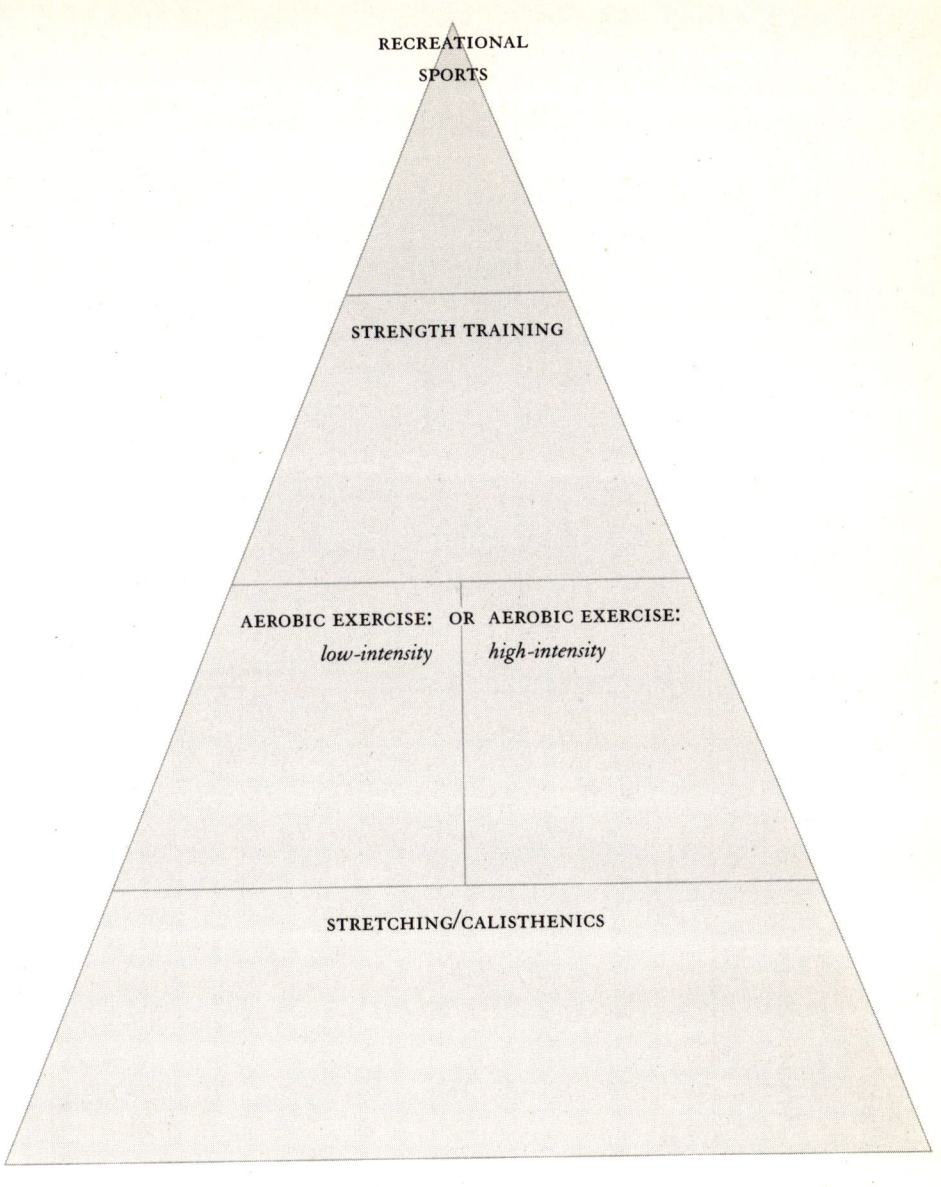

Exercise Diary Pyramid
Make photocopies of this page and use it to record the types and amount of exercise you get each day (refer back to the appropriate exercise pyramid in chapter 13 to remind yourself of the appropriate exercise program for your risk level). You can also use the blank pyramid to help you plan an exercise program that fulfills your goals.

Weekly Exercise Diary

week starting: _____ ending: _____

risk level: _____	Aerobic exercise	Strength-Building Exercise	Stretching/Calisthenics	Recreational Sports
Monday				
Tuesday				
Wednesday				
Thursday				
Friday				
Saturday				
Sunday				

Supplement Diary for Level 1: Prevention

DATE: _____

Supplement	Dosage per Pill	Number of Pills Taken		
		Breakfast	Lunch	Dinner
Multivitamin and mineral complex				

Supplement Diary for Level 2: Low Risk

DATE: _____

SUPPLEMENT	DOSAGE	TIME OF DAY TAKEN		
		BREAKFAST	LUNCH	DINNER
MULTIVITAMIN AND MINERAL COMPLEX				
VITAMIN C (BUFFERED)				
VITAMIN E: MIXED TOCOPHEROLS TOCOTRIENOLS				
VITAMIN B-COMPLEX				
CALCIUM AND MAGNESIUM				
ESSENTIAL FATTY ACIDS (EPA AND DHA)				

Supplement Diary for Level 3: Moderate Risk

DATE: _____

SUPPLEMENT	DOSAGE PER PILL	NUMBER OF PILLS TAKEN		
		BREAKFAST	LUNCH	DINNER
MULTIVITAMIN AND MINERAL COMPLEX				
VITAMIN C (BUFFERED)				
VITAMIN E: MIXED TOCOPHEROLS TOCOTRIENOLS				
VITAMIN B-COMPLEX				
CALCIUM AND MAGNESIUM				
ESSENTIAL FATTY ACIDS (EPA AND DHA)				
NIACIN				
ARGININE				
COENZYME Q_{10}				
GUGGULIPID				
POLICOSANOL				
RED YEAST RICE				

Supplement Diary for Level 4: High Risk

DATE: _____

Supplement	Dosage per pill	Number of Pills Taken		
		Breakfast	Lunch	Dinner
Multivitamin and mineral complex				
Vitamin C (buffered)				
Vitamin E: mixed tocopherols tocotrienols				
Vitamin B-complex				
Calcium and magnesium				
Essential fatty acids (EPA and DHA)				
Niacin				
Arginine				
Coenzyme Q_{10}				
Guggulipid				

	Policosanol	Red yeast rice	Alpha-lipoic acid	Bromelain	Turmeric (curcumin)	Ginkgo	Garlic	Grapeseed extract	Hawthorn	L-Carnitine	Milk thistle	Pantethine	Taurine			

Stress and Relaxation Diary

This diary format is just a suggestion for how you can keep a log of your daily sources of stress and your daily sources of relaxation. As I mentioned in chapter 14, you will need to modify this template to your unique style of expression. If you are extremely time-conscious, well-organized, and precise, a daily log based around time and activity, utilizing bullets and short sentences, might be appropriate for you. You can carry your log around with you and fill in activities and feelings as you go through your day. If you have no opportunity to do this, or if your mind works in an associative rather than a linear fashion, you may prefer to take some quiet time at the end of each day, or during your lunch hour, to reflect on the day's stressors and perks. Once again, I recommend photocopying the blank pages and using the photocopies to create your personal record.

Stress and Relaxation Diary

DATE: _____

Time of Day	Activity	Feeling

TODAY'S STRESSORS:

TODAY'S PERKS:

AREAS TO WORK ON:

# 17 Conclusions

To repair the world...
—Ancient Jewish prayer

Despite the exciting scientific advances on the horizon, cardiovascular disease remains the leading cause of death worldwide. Heart disease and stroke killed 17 million people in the year 1999—about 30 percent of all deaths. This figure represents a significant and extremely disturbing increase, compared to the 14.7 million deaths reported in 1990. In a September 2000 editorial that appeared in *Circulation: Journal of the American Heart Association*, Dr. Bonow wrote, "We must do a more effective job of translating scientific advances into programs that can save lives in all parts of the world."

The editorial was written in conjunction with World Heart Day (September 29, 2000), sponsored by the World Heart Federation, a Geneva-based organization. The focus of World Heart Day was on establishing a healthy lifestyle, including healthier eating and increased exercise. In fact, Global Embrace, the annual advocacy event of the

Global Movement for Active Ageing, coordinated its main events to coincide with World Heart Day, and with the International Day of Older Persons. In 2002, they made walking the prime focus of their events. In the words of Dr. Gro Harlem Brundtland, director-general of the World Health Organization, "We have an immediate, safe and reliable remedy [to reduce] some of the major health risks linked to unhealthy consumption. It is free. It works for rich and poor, for men and women, for young and old. It is physical activity."

Preventing heart disease is completely viable and realistic, but requires a holistic approach. It involves looking at areas of lifestyle that have an impact on physical health—exercise, diet, and stress—and making heart-healthy changes when necessary in these areas. It also means learning to love yourself in an entirely different way. Implementing the DEAR program and the CARE diet are concrete ways to create a health-producing, self-loving lifestyle. And remember that this type of self-love isn't selfish. On the contrary, the greatest gift you can give to others is your own health and vitality. When you feel well and vigorous, you are in a much better position to share yourself and your love with family, friends, your community, and the entire global community. When you are ill, your effectiveness, energy level, and strength can be compromised, and often, others must take care of you. Moreover, when you feel happy and strong, you become a role model for others. People want to know what your secret is. Sharing you wisdom and experiences with others can teach them how to take better care of themselves as well.

There is an ancient Jewish Kabbalistic concept called *tikkum olam*—the repair of the world. Human actions should ideally be undertaken with this goal of planetary healing in mind. Self-healing and self-love contribute to global healing and universal love. I wish you healing and love as you embark upon your journey toward optimum health, and I wish you many opportunities to share your health with others.

Glossary

adhesion molecules. Substances released by the intimal layer in response to injury, such as the infiltration of LDL cholesterol, making the endothelial surface sticky and adhesive.

advanced, complicated atherosclerotic lesion. The building block of plaque, this is a deposit under the endothelium and in the intima consisting of fat-filled macrophages, immune factors, and debris and covered by a fibrous cap consisting of smooth muscles.

adventitia. The outer layer of the blood vessel.

aerobic exercise. Exercises such as walking, jogging, or swimming in which the body moves consistently in a regular rhythm, producing maximum utilization of oxygen.

amino acids. The building blocks of proteins. Nine of the basic amino acids are essential, meaning that the body cannot manufacture them and therefore they must be obtained from food.

angina pectoris. A condition caused by the narrowing of arteries, thereby preventing sufficient blood flow to the heart. The most common symptom is chest pain or tightness, especially during exertion.

angioplasty. The use of a balloonlike device to compress plaque against arterial walls, thereby widening the space of the lumen. Also called *ballooning*.

aorta. A large artery that is the main trunk of the body's arterial system, arising from the left ventricle of the heart.

apoprotein. A protein that transports lipids through the bloodstream. When it combines with a lipid, it's called a lipoprotein.

arrhythmia. Irregular heartbeat.

atherosclerosis. Hardening of the arteries due to plaque buildup. Plaque deposits prevent the arterial walls from expanding and contracting as they should.

body mass index (BMI). A calculation of your height and weight that indicates whether you are overweight. If your weight is correct for your height, you have a normal BMI. If you are overweight, your BMI will be elevated.

bypass surgery. A surgical procedure redirecting blood flow around a blocked artery, using part of a blood vessel taken from another part of the body.

capillaries. The tiniest blood vessels through which the blood delivers oxygen and nutrients to the cells.

cholesterol. An odorless, waxy substance manufactured in our liver and from fat that we get in our diets. Some cholesterol is necessary to maintain good health, but too much cholesterol (especially LDL cholesterol) is destructive because it contributes to atherosclerosis.

congestive heart failure. A condition that occurs when the heart is unable to pump sufficient blood, due to weakness or dysfunctional valves, leading to fluid buildup around the lungs and often in other parts of the body. Typical symptoms include shortness of breath and congestion in the lungs, or swelling in the lower extremities, such as the ankles.

coronary arteries. Arteries that branch off the aorta and supply blood to the heart.

coronary artery disease. Narrowing of the coronary arteries, usually caused by plaque, leading to heart attack or angina. Sometimes also called *coronary heart disease*.

C-reactive protein (CRP). A protein that increases when inflammation is present. Because it is a marker of inflammation, it is being used to measure the risk of cardiovascular disease, now understood to be an inflammatory process. While C–reactive protein measures all types of inflammation, the type of CRP most closely associated with cardiovascular disease is called *cardiac CRP* or *high-sensitivity CRP (hs-CRP)*.

cytokines. Naturally occurring chemical messengers that affect inflammation and the immune system.

diastole. Relaxation of the heart, allowing the return of blood.

endothelial derived relaxing factor (EDRF). A substance released by the endothelium, containing nitric oxide. It is responsible for the relaxation and expansion of the blood vessel walls.

endothelial dysfunction. Malfunction of the endothelium, involving a widening of the gaps between endothelial cells, allowing invaders to penetrate the intima. A dysfunctional endothelium is unable to expand and contract properly.

endothelium. The lining of cells that covers the inner layer of blood vessels.

fatty streak. The earliest sign of atherosclerotic plaque.

fibrinogen. A blood protein necessary for proper clotting. Elevated fibrinogen makes the blood too sticky and prone to clotting.

foam cells. Fat-filled macrophages within the intimal layer. Foam cells are the basic building blocks of a plaque lesion.

free radicals. Chemicals consisting of a molecule with an unpaired electron. These electrons scavenge and "kidnap" electrons from molecules in the body's cells, causing damage.

heart attack. See *myocardial infarction.*

hemoglobin. A naturally occurring substance made largely of iron and mixed with protein and other substances. It is responsible for giving red blood cells their color.

high-density lipoprotein (HDL cholesterol). This type of cholesterol (commonly called "good") confers protective benefit on the blood vessels.

HMG-CoA reductase inhibitors. See *statins.*

homeostasis. Balance and status quo.

homocysteine. A by-product of the breakdown of an amino acid called methionine. Because elevated levels of homocysteine are associated with increased risk of cardiovascular disease, homocysteine has become incorporated into blood tests that screen for cardiovascular risk factors.

hypertension. High blood pressure, an established risk factor for cardiovascular disease.

inflammation. A group of chemical changes produced by the body's immune system as a response to injury or abnormal stimulation inflicted by a physical, chemical, or biological agent.

intermittent claudication. Pain in the legs during walking or exertion due to peripheral artery disease.

intima. The inner layer of the blood vessel.

ischemia. A condition in which blood flow to the heart is reduced. It is typically caused by narrowing of the coronary blood vessels. Also called *cardiac insufficiency.*

leukocyte. A type of white blood cell involved in the immune process.

lipid. Fatty substance in our body.

lipoprotein. The combination of a lipid and an apoprotein.

lipoprotein (a) (Lp[a]). A protein contained in cholesterol that plays a role in blood clotting. Elevated Lp(a) is a serious risk factor for the development of cardiovascular disease.

low-density lipoprotein (LDL cholesterol). Often called the "bad" cholesterol, this type of cholesterol infiltrates the endothelium and leads to the buildup of plaque.

lumen. The channel within the blood vessel through which the blood flows.

macrophages. Immune cells that "gobble" fat globules within the intima. They are the mature form of monocytes.

media. The middle layer of the blood vessel.

monocytes. Immune cells sent to the site of a cholesterol deposit in the intima.

myocardial infarction. Commonly known as a heart attack, this occurs when a blockage in the artery prevents blood flow to the heart, and some cardiac tissue dies as a result. Symptoms of heart attack are chest pain, often radiating into the arms or jaw; heavy feeling in the chest; shortness of breath; feeling of unease; or nausea.

necrosis. Decay caused by the death of tissue.

nitric oxide. A chemical present in EDRF that plays a role in the relaxation and expansion of blood vessel walls.

oxidized and modified cholesterol. When an LDL cholesterol molecule is within the intima, it combines with oxygen to form oxidized cholesterol. This new compound, in turn, combines with sugar particles to form modified cholesterol.

peripheral artery disease. Hardening of the arteries in the legs, leading to intermittent claudication.

plaque. Buildup of cholesterol, immune cells, and debris under the endothelial wall of the artery. Plaque buildup is responsible for atherosclerosis.

platelets. Clotting agents in the blood. They are responsible for stickiness and clumping together of blood after injury.

remodeling. The reshaping of the lumen to accommodate the plaque lesion.

restenosis. Renarrowing of an artery following angioplasty or bypass surgery.

smooth muscle cells. Cells contained in the middle layer of the blood vessel (which is made of smooth muscles) that migrate to cover foam cells and seal them off by forming a fibrous "cap."

stable plaque. Plaque covered by a firm, solid fibrous cap consisting of smooth muscle and connective tissue.

statins. Medications designed to reduce cholesterol levels and recently discovered to also have an anti-inflammatory effect. They have been associated with serious side effects, including liver dysfunction, muscular pain, fatigue, numbness, tingling, memory loss, and, in a few individuals, a disease called rhabdomyolysis. Also called *HMG-CoA reductase inhibitors*.

stent. A cagelike device inserted during angioplasty to hold the lumen open.

stroke. Also called cerebral vascular accident, this occurs when an artery is blocked, preventing blood flow to the brain, or when a blood vessel in the brain ruptures. Symptoms include sudden weakness, numbness, tingling, or loss of vision (especially affecting only one side); dizziness or disorientation; difficulty speaking; or sudden intense headache.

syndrome X. A cluster of risk factors for cardiovascular disease often appearing together and working synergistically to increase the overall risk. These include hypertension, diabetes, obesity, elevated LDL cholesterol, low HDL cholesterol, and elevated triglycerides.

systole. The pumping, contracting phase of cardiac activity that forces blood out of the heart and into the arteries.

thrombus. Blood clot.

T-lymphocytes. A type of white blood cell involved in the immune response.

transient ischemic attack. Commonly called a "mini-stroke," this is similar to a stroke, but its symptoms last for shorter periods of time. Often, it precedes a stroke.

triglycerides. Fats manufactured in the liver or derived from food and used by the body as a source of energy. When not being used, they are stored. Elevated triglycerides are a major risk factor for CVD and also signal insulin resistance, which can be a precursor for diabetes.

type A personality. A person who is intensely ambitious, driven, anxious, tense, and perfectionistic. These traits are associated with a higher risk of cardiovascular disease.

unstable plaque. A plaque lesion whose fibrous cap is eroded or in the process of thinning out and therefore is prone to rupture. Also called *vulnerable plaque*.

valvular heart disease. A narrowing or leakage in one or more of the heart's valves.

very low-density lipoprotein (VLDL). The lipoprotein unit that transports triglycerides.

vulnerable plaque. See *unstable plaque*.

white blood cells. Cells present in the bloodstream that are responsible for the immune response.

Suggestions for Further Reading

Alter, Judy. *Stretch and Strengthen*. Boston: Houghton Mifflin, 1986.

American Lung Association, Edwin B. Fisher, Jr., Everett Koop. *American Lung Association, 7 Steps to a Smoke-Free Life*. New York: John Wiley and Sons, Inc., 1998.

Balch, Phyllis A., and James F. Balch. *Prescription for Nutritional Healing*, 3rd ed. New York: Avery/Penguin/Putnam, 2002.

Benson, Herbert. *The Relaxation Response*. New York: Morrow/Avon Books, 2000.

Borysenko, Joan. *Minding the Body, Mending the Mind*. Reading, MA: Addison-Wesley, 1987.

Bratman, Steven, and Richard Harkness. *Drug-Herb-Vitamin Interactions Bible*. Rosemont, CA: Prima Publishing, 2001.

Challem, Jack, Burton Berkson, and Melissa Diane Smith. *Syndrome X*. New York: John Wiley and Sons, Inc., 2000.

Cohen, Jay. *Over Dose: The Case Against the Drug Companies*. New York: Jeremy P. Tarcher/Putnam, 2001.

Cooke, John P., and Judith Zimmer. *The Cardiovascular Cure*. New York: Broadway Books, 2002.

Cooper, Kenneth. *Overcoming Hypertension*. New York: Bantam Books, 1990.

Hilleman, Richard. *Richard Hilleman's Yoga 28 Day Exercise Plan*. New York: Bantam Books, 1969.

Hooton, Claire. *Tai Chi for Beginners: Ten Minutes of Health and Fitness*. New York: Berkley Books, 1996.

Kabat-Zinn, Jon. *Full Catastrophe Living.* New York: Delta Books, 1990.

———. *Mindfulness Meditation: Cultivating the Wisdom of Your Body and Mind* (audiocassette). Niles, IL: Nightingale Conant, 1995.

———. *Wherever You Go, There You Are: Mindfulness Meditation in Everyday Life.* New York: Hyperion, 1995.

Kaptchuk, Ted. *The Web That Has No Weaver: Understanding Chinese Medicine.* Lincolnwood, IL: NTC/Contemporary Publishing, 2000.

Karony, Stephenie, and Anthony L. Ranken. *Workouts with Weights: Simple Routines You Can Do at Home.* New York: Sterling Publishing Company, 1993.

Janson, Michael. *The Vitamin Revolution in Health Care.* Greenville, NH: Arcadia Press, 1996.

LeShan, Lawrence. *How to Meditate.* New York: Bantam Books, 1984.

Levine, Peter A. *Waking the Tiger: Healing Trauma.* Berkeley, CA: North Atlantic Books, 1997.

Lieberman, Shari. *Get Off the Menopause Roller Coaster.* New York: Avery/Penguin/Putnam, 2000.

———. *The Real Vitamin and Mineral Book.* Garden City Park, NY: Avery Publishing Group, 1997.

Lingerman, Hal A. *The Healing Energies of Music.* Wheaton, IL: Quest Books, 1983.

Lininger, Schuyler Jr., ed. *The A–Z Guide to Drug-Herb and Vitamin Interactions.* Rosemont, CA: Prima Publishing, 1999.

Lipson, Elaine Marie. *The Organic Foods Source Book.* New York: Contemporary Books, 2001.

Magaziner, Allan. *The Complete Idiot's Guide to Living Longer and Healthier.* New York: Alpha Books, 1999.

———. *The Total Health Handbook: Your Complete Wellness Resource.* New York: Kensington Books, 2000.

Magaziner, Allan, Linda Bonvie, and Anthony Zolezzi. *Chemical-Free Kids: How to Safeguard Your Child's Diet and Environment.* New York: Kensington Books, 2003.

Natow, Annette B., and Jo-Ann Heslin. *The Most Complete Food Counter.* New York: Pocket Books, 1999.

Northrup, Christiane. *The Wisdom of Menopause: Creating Physical and Emotional Health and Healing During the Change.* New York: Bantam, Doubleday, Dell, 2001.

Rothfeld, Glenn, and Suzanne Levert. *The Acupuncture Response*. New York: Contemporary Books, 2002.

Schiffman, Erich. *Yoga—The Spirit and Practice of Moving into Stillness*. New York: Simon and Schuster, 1996.

Schleck, Lorie A., ed. *Staying Strong: A Senior's Guide to a More Active and Independent Life*. Minneapolis: Fairview Press, 2000.

Shapiro, Francine, and Margot Silk Forrest. *EMDR: The Breakthrough Therapy for Overcoming Anxiety, Stress and Trauma*. New York: Basic Books, 1998.

Shimer, Porter. *Too Busy to Exercise*. Pownal, VT: Barnes and Noble Books, 2000.

Siegel, Bernie. *Love, Medicine and Miracles*. New York: Harper and Row, 1986.

———. *Peace, Love and Healing*. New York: Harper and Row, 1989.

Sinatra, Stephen T., Jan Sinatra, and Roberta Jo Lieberman. *Heart Sense for Women*. New York: Penguin/Plume, 2000.

Sloan, Jim. *Staying Fit Over 50—Conditioning for Outdoor Activities*. Seattle: The Mountaineers, 1999.

Solomon, Neil, Rita Elkins, and Richard Passwater. *Soy Smart Health*. Pleasant Grove, UT: Woodland Publishing, 2000.

Ward, Susan Winter. *Yoga for the Young at Heart: Gentle Stretching Exercises for Seniors*. Santa Barbara, CA: Capra Press, 1994.

Westcott, Wayne L., and Thomas Baechle. *Strength Training for Seniors*. Champaign, IL: Human Kinetics Publications, 1995.

Selected References

Allen, Jane E. "An Oral History." *Los Angeles Times.* 8 March 1999.

Anderson, K. J., S. S. Teuber, A. Gobeille, et al. "Walnut polyphenolics inhibit in vitro human plasma and LDL oxidation." *Journal of Nutrition.* 2001;131:2837–42.

Ansell, B. J. "Should physicians be recommending statins for most older Americans?" *Clinical Geriatrics.* 2002;10:33–40.

Aviram, M., and B. Fuhrman. "Wine flavonoids protect against LDL oxidation and atherosclerosis." *Ann. N.Y. Acad. Sci.* 2002;957:146–61.

Beckman, J. A., M. A. Creager, and P. Libby. "Diabetes and atherosclerosis: epidemiology, pathophysiology, and management." *JAMA.* 2002;287:2570–81.

Berenson, G. S. "Childhood risk factors predict adult risk associated with subclinical cardiovascular disease: the Bogalusa Heart Study." *Am J Cardiol.* 2002;90:3L–7L.

Brosse, A. L., E. S. Sheets, H. S. Lett, et al. "Exercise and the treatment of clinical depression in adults: recent findings and future directions." *Sports Med.* 2002;32:741–60.

Colodny, L. R., A. Montgomery, and M. Houston. "The role of esterin-processed alfalfa saponins in reducing cholesterol." *JAMA.* 2001;3:6–15.

Danesh, J., P. Whincup, M. Walker, et al. "Low-grade inflammation and coronary heart disease: prospective study and updated meta-analyses." *BMJ.* 2000;321:199–204.

Davi, G., M. T. Guagnano, G. Ciabattoni, et al. "Platelet activation in obese women: role of inflammation and oxidant stress." *JAMA.* 2002;288:2006–14.

DiLoreto, S. "Using drugs to prevent CVD in high-risk patients." *Patient Care.* 2001;40–55.

Djurhuus, M. S., N. A. Klitgaard, K. K. Pedersen, et al. "Magnesium reduces insulin-stimulated glucose uptake and serum lipid concentrations in type 1 diabetes." *Metabolism.* 2001;50:1409–17.

Fairfield, K. M., and R. H. Fletcher. "Vitamins for chronic disease prevention in adults: scientific review." *JAMA.* 2002;287:3116–26.

Falkenberg, Lisa. "High Triglycerides are called a Stroke Predictor." *Philadelphia Inquirer.* 11 Dec 2001.

Farmer, J. A. "Lipid-lowering therapy in patients with hypertension." *Lipid Management.* 2003;8.

Fichtlscherer, S., G. Rosenberger, D. H. Walter, et al. "Elevated C-reactive protein levels and impaired endothelial vasoreactivity in patients with coronary artery disease." *Circulation.* 2000;102:1000.

Fignar, J. M. "Rhabdomyolysis: a clinical syndrome." *Journal of the POMA.* 2002;15–17, 37.

Fitzpatrick, A. "Conventional and natural therapies for hyperlipidemia." *International Journal of Integrative Medicine.* 2002;4:8–18.

Flegal, K. M., M. D. Carroll, C. L. Ogden, et al. "Prevalence and trends in obesity among US adults, 1999–2000." *JAMA.* 2002;288:1723–32.

Fletcher, R. H., and K. M. Fairfield. "Vitamins for chronic disease prevention in adults: clinical applications." *JAMA.* 2002;287:3127–29.

Fletcher, S. W. "Failure of estrogen plus progestin therapy for prevention." *JAMA.* 2002;288:366–67.

Fox, C., D. Ramsoomair, and C. Carter. "Magnesium: its proven and potential clinical significance." *South Med J.* 2001;94:1195–1201.

Fraser, G. E., H. W. Bennett, K. B. Jaceldo, et al. "Effect on body weight of a free 76 kilojoule (320 calorie) daily supplement of almonds for six months." *Journal of the American College of Nutrition.* 2002;21:275–83.

Fuhrman, B., N. Volkova, M. Kaplan, et al. "Antiatherosclerotic effects of licorice extract supplementation on hypercholesterolemic patients: increased resistance of LDL to atherogenic modifications, reduced plasma lipid levels, and decreased systolic blood pressure." *Nutrition.* 2002;18:268–73.

Garcia, R. I., E. A. Krall, and P. S. Vokonas. "Periodontal disease and mortality from all causes in the VA Dental Longitudinal Study." *Annals of Periodontology.* 1998;3:339–49.

Goldstein, J. A., D. Demetriou, C. L. Grines, et al. "Multiple complex coronary plaques in patients with acute myocardial infarction." *N Eng J Med.* 2000;343:915.

Greenland, P., M. D. Knoll, J. Stamler, et al. "Major risk factors as antecedents of fatal and nonfatal coronary heart disease events." *JAMA.* 2003;290:891–97.

Hackam, D. G., and S. S. Anand. "Emerging risk factors for atherosclerotic vascular disease: a critical review of the evidence." *JAMA.* 2003;290:932–40.

Hamilton-Craig, I. "Statin-associated myopathy." *Med J Aust.* 2001;175:486–89.

He, K., E. B. Rimm, A. Merchant, et al. "Fish consumption and risk of stroke in men." *JAMA.* 2002;288:3130.

Heber, D., I. Yip, J. M. Ashley, et al. "Cholesterol-lowering effects of a proprietary Chinese red-yeast-rice dietary supplement." *Am J Clin Nutr.* 1999;69:231–36.

Hines, S. E. "Do antioxidants prevent heart disease?" *Patient Care.* 2000;72–73.

Howard, B. V., and D. Kritchevsky. "Phytochemicals and cardiovascular disease: a statement for healthcare professionals from the American Heart Association." *Circulation.* 1997;95:2591–93.

Hu, F. B., J. E. Manson, and W. C. Willett. "Types of dietary fat and risk of coronary heart disease: a critical review." *Journal of the American College of Nutrition.* 2001;20:5–19.

Hu, F. B., and W. C. Willett. "Optimal diets for prevention of coronary heart disease." *JAMA.* 2002;288:2569–78.

Iannuzzi, A., E. Celentano, S. Panico, et al. "Dietary and circulating antioxidant vitamins in relation to carotid plaques in middle-aged women." *Am J Clin Nutr.* 2002;76:582.

Irwin, M. L., Y. Yasui, C. M. Ulrich, et al. "Effects of exercise on total and intra-abdominal body fat in postmenopausal women: a randomized controlled trial." *JAMA.* 2003;289:323–30.

Jancin, B. "Cholesterol Guidelines 'Hopelessly Out of Date.'" *Family Practice News.* 15 June 2003.

Jenkins, D. J. A., C. W. C. Kendall, A. Marchie, et al. "Effects of a dietary portfolio of cholesterol-lowering foods vs lovastatin on serum lipids and C-reactive protein." *JAMA.* 2003;290:502–10.

Jiang, R., J. E. Manson, M. J. Stampfer, et al. "Nut and peanut butter consumption and risk of type 2 diabetes in women." *JAMA.* 2002;288:2554–60.

Kawamoto, R., T. Kajiwara, Y. Oka, et al. "Association between abdominal wall fat index and carotid atherosclerosis in women." *J Atheroscler Thromb.* 2002; 9:213–18.

Khosh, F., and M. Khosh. "Natural approach to hypertension." *Alternative Medicine Review.* 2001;6:590–600.

Krueger, P. M. "Hormone replacement therapy: guiding our patients through WHI and HERS." *The Journal.* 2002;6–8.

Kumar, B., M. N. Jha, and W. C. Cole. "D-alpha-Tocopheryl Succinate (vitamin E) enhances radiation-induced chromosomal damage levels in human cancer cells, but reduces it in normal cells." *Journal of the American College of Nutrition.* 2002;21:339–43.

Lacey, J. V. "Menopausal hormone replacement therapy and risk of ovarian cancer." *JAMA.* 2002;288:334–41.

Law, M. R., and J. K. Morris. "By how much does fruit and vegetable consumption reduce the risk of ischaemic heart disease?" *European Journal of Clinical Nutrition.* 1998;52:549–56.

Lemonick, Michael D. "Rethinking a Heart-Disease Risk." *Time.* 4 Nov 2002, 109.

Libby, P., and P. M. Ridker. "Novel inflammatory markers of coronary risk: theory versus practice." *Circulation.* 1999;100:1148–50.

Lucas, K. H. "Herbal products: pearls, perils, and precautions for the prescriber." *The Female Patient.* 2002;27:45–49.

Maxwell, A. J., B. E. Anderson, and J. P. Cooke. "Nutritional therapy for peripheral arterial disease: a double-blind, placebo-controlled, randomized trial of Heartbar." *Vasc Med.* 2000, 5:11–19.

Maxwell, A. J., M. P. Zapien, G. L. Pearce, et al. "Randomized trial of a medical food for the dietary management of chronic, stable angina." *J Am Coll Cardiol.* 2002;39:37–45.

McKay, D. L., and J. B. Blumberg. "The role of tea in human health: an update." *Journal of the American College of Nutrition.* 2002;21:1–13.

Mendez, M. V., T. Scott, W. LaMorte, et al. "An association between periodontal disease and peripheral vascular disease." *The American Journal of Surgery.* 1998;176:153–57.

Mercola, J. "Just one extra serving of vegetables lowers heart disease." *Annals of Internal Medicine.* 2001;134:1106–14.

Moon, M. A. "CRP may Predict Cardio Events Better than LDL Levels." *Family Practice News.* 1 Jan 2003.

Morelli, V., and R. J. Zoorob. "Alternative therapies: Part II. Congestive heart failure and hypercholesterolemia." *Am Fam Physician.* 2000;62:1051–60.

Nash, D. T. "Keeping an eye on cardiovascular risk: a practical, case-study approach to assessment in office practice." *Postgraduate Medicine.* 2002;111:107–20.

Neumann, F. J., A. Kastrati, T. Miethke, et al. "Previous cytomegalovirus infection and risk of coronary thrombotic events after stent placement." *Circulation.* 2000;101:11.

Newby, L. K., A. Kristinsson, M. V. Bhapkar, et al. "Early statin initiation and outcomes in patients with acute coronary syndromes." *JAMA.* 2002;287:3087–95.

Nied, R. J., and B. Franklin. "Promoting and prescribing exercise for the elderly." *Am Fam Physician.* 2002;65:419–26.

Nielsen, S. J., and B. M. Popkin. "Patterns and trends in food portion sizes, 1977–1998." *JAMA.* 2003;289:450–53.

Noller, K. L. "Estrogen replacement therapy and risk of ovarian cancer." *JAMA.* 2002;288:368–69.

Ogden, C. L., K. M. Flegal, M. D. Carroll, et al. "Prevalence and trends in overweight among US children and adolescents, 1999–2000." *JAMA.* 2002;288:1728–32.

Omar, M. A., J. P. Wilson, and T. S. Cox. "Rhabdomyolysis and HMG-CoA reductase inhibitors." *Ann Pharmacother.* 2001;35:1096–1107.

Patrick, L., and M. Uzick. "Cardiovascular disease: C-reactive protein and the inflammatory disease paradigm: HMG-CoA reductase inhibitors, alpha-tocopherol, red yeast rice, and olive oil polyphenols. A review of the literature." *Alternative Medicine Review.* 2001;6:248–71.

Pennachio, D. L. "Strategies for maintaining heart health." *Patient Care.* 2001; 56–64.

Rao, A. V., and S. Agarwal. "Role of antioxidant lycopene in cancer and heart disease." *Journal of the American College of Nutrition.* 2000;19:563–69.

———. "Role of lycopene as antioxidant carotenoid in the prevention of chronic diseases: a review." *Nutrition Research.* 1999;19:305–23.

Reddy, M. S., and S. C. Gupta. "Diabetes and cardiovascular disease: two cardiologists review the effects of diabetes on the cardiovascular system, the influence of these effects on morbidity and mortality risks, and how to incorporate these special considerations into the management of patients in primary care." *Emergency Medicine.* 2002;28–35.

Ridker, P. M., M. Cushman, M. J. Stampfer, et al. "Inflammation, aspirin, and the risk of cardiovascular disease in apparently healthy men." *N Engl J Med.* 1997;336:973–79.

Ridker, P. M., C. H. Hennekens, J. E. Buring, et al. "C-reactive protein and other markers of inflammation in the prediction of cardiovascular disease in women." *N Engl J Med.* 2000;342:836–43.

Ridker, P. M., N. Rifai, M. Clearfield, et al. "Measurement of C-reactive protein for the targeting of statin therapy in the primary prevention of acute coronary events." *N Engl J Med.* 2001;344:1959.

Ridker, P. M., N. Rifai, L. Rose, et al. "Comparison of C-reactive protein and low-density lipoprotein cholesterol levels in the prediction of first cardiovascular events." *N Engl J Med.* 2002;347:1557–65.

Ridker, P. M., M. J. Stampfer, and N. Rifai. "Novel risk factors for systemic atherosclerosis: a comparison of C-reactive protein, fibrinogen, homocysteine, lipoprotein(a), and standard cholesterol screening as predictors of peripheral arterial disease." *JAMA.* 2001;285:2481–85.

Sabaté, J., G. E. Fraser, K. Burke, et al. "Effects of walnuts on serum lipid levels and blood pressure in normal men." *N Engl J Med.* 1993;328:603–607.

Safeer, R. S., and P. S. Ugalat. "Cholesterol treatment guidelines update." *Am Fam Physician.* 2002;65:871–80.

Schnyder, G., M. Roffi, Y. Flammer, et al. "Effect of homocysteine-lowering therapy with folic acid, vitamin B_{12}, and vitamin B_6 on clinical outcome after percutaneous coronary intervention: the Swiss Heart Study: a randomized controlled trial." *JAMA.* 2002;288:973–79.

Sessa, R., M. Di Pietro, I. Santino, et al. "Chlamydia pneumoniae infection and atherosclerotic coronary disease." *Am Heart J.* 1999;137:1116–19.

Shechter, M., M. Sharir, M. J. Labrador, et al. "Oral magnesium therapy improves endothelial function in patients with coronary artery disease." *Circulation.* 2000;102:2353–58.

Sheetz, M. J., and G. L. King. "Molecular understanding of hyperglycemia's adverse effects for diabetic complications." *JAMA.* 2002;288:2579–88.

Sica, D. A., and T. W. Gehr. "Rhabdomyolysis and statin therapy: relevance to the elderly." *Am J Geriatr Cardiol.* 2002;11:48–55.

Siscovick, D. S., S. M. Schwartz, L. Corey, et al. "Chlamydia pneumoniae, herpes simplex virus type 1, and cytomegalovirus and incident myocardial infarction and coronary heart disease death in older adults." *Circulation.* 2000;102:2335.

Slavkin, H. C., and B. J. Baum. "Relationship of dental and oral pathology to systemic illness." *JAMA.* 2000;284:1215–17.

Stewart, K. J. "Exercise training and the cardiovascular consequences of type 2 diabetes and hypertension: plausible mechanisms for improving cardiovascular health." *JAMA.* 202;288:1622–31.

Strawbridge, W. J., S. Deleger, R. E. Roberts, et al. "Physical activity reduces the risk of subsequent depression for older adults." *Am J Epidemio.* 2002;156:328–34.

Sullivan, M. G. "Treat Syndrome X with Whole Foods Eating Plan." *Family Practice News*. 15 Jan 2003.

Tomeo, A. C., M. Geller, T. R. Watkins, et al. "Antioxidant effects of tocotrienols in patients with hyperlipidemia and carotid stenosis." *Lipids*. 1995;30:1179–83.

Tomlinson, B., P. Chan, and W. Lan. "How well tolerated are lipid-lowering drugs?" *Drugs Aging*. 2001;18:665–83.

Williams, C. L., L. L. Hayman, S. R. Daniels, et al. "Cardiovascular health in childhood: a statement for health professionals from the committee on Atherosclerosis, Hypertension, and Obesity in the Young (AHOY) of the Council on Cardiovascular Disease in the Young, American Heart Association." *Circulation*. 2002;106:143–60.

Wink, J., G. Giacoppe, and J. King. "Effect of very-low-dose niacin on high-density lipoprotein in patients undergoing long-term statin therapy." *Am Heart J*. 2002;143:514–18.

Zoler, M. L. "Heart Association Advocates Fish Oil Supplements." *Family Practice News*. 15 Jan 2003.

Resources

Throughout this book, I have promised you information about how to obtain various types of products or services. It is not possible to give an exhaustive list, of course, but this section contains some excellent leads to get you started. Please remember that contact information for organizations is subject to change.

SPECIFIC HEALTH ISSUES

American Diabetes Association
(ATTN: National Call Center)
1701 North Beauregard Street
Alexandria, VA 22311
800-DIABETES (800-342-2383)
www.diabetes.org

American Heart Association
American Stroke Association
7320 Greenville Avenue
Dallas, TX 75321
888-AHA-USA-1 (888-242-8721) for heart-related information
888-4-STROKE (888-478-7653) for stroke-related information
www.americanheart.org

American Lung Association
212-315-8700
www.lungusa.org

American Obesity Association
1250 24th Street NW, Suite 300
Washington, DC 20037
212-776-7711
www.obesity.org

American Psychological Association
202-336-3500
800-324-2721
www.apa.org

American Society of Hypertension
148 Madison Avenue, 5th Floor
New York, NY 10016
212-696-9099
www.ash-us.org

Center for Science in the Public Interest (Food Safety)
1875 Connecticut Avenue NW, Suite 300
Washington, DC 20009-5728
202-332-9110
www.cspinet.org

Food and Nutrition Information Center
Agricultural Research Service, USDA
National Agricultural Library, Room 105
10301 Baltimore Avenue
Beltsville, MD 20705-2351
301-504-1719
TTY: 301-504-6856
www.nal.usda.gov/fnic/

Overeaters Anonymous
505-891-2664
www.overeatersanonymous.org

REFERRAL SOURCES FOR ALTERNATIVE, COMPLEMENTARY, AND INTEGRATIVE MEDICINE PRACTITIONERS

American Academy of Environmental Medicine
316-684-5500
www.aaem.com

American Academy of Medical Acupuncture
323-937-5514
www.medicalacupuncture.org

American Academy of Periodontology
312-573-3243
www.perio.org

American Art Therapy Association
888-290-0878
www.arttherapy.org

American Association of Naturopathic Physicians
866-538-2267
www.naturopathic.org

American Association of Oriental Medicine (AAOM)
888-500-7999
E-mail: aaom1@aol.com

American College for Advancement in Medicine
800-532-3688
www.acam.org

American Dance Therapy Association
410-997-4040
www.adta.org

American Herb Association
P.O. Box 1673
Nevada City, CA 95959
530-265-9552
www.ahaherb.com

American Herbalists Guild
P.O. Box 746555
Arvada, CO 80006
303-423-8800
www.wvu.edu

American Holistic Medical Association
505-202-7788
www.ahma.org

American Holistic Nurses Association
800-278-2462
www.ahna.org/

American Massage Therapy Association
847-864-0123
www.amtamassage.org

American Music Therapy Association
301-589-3300
www.musictherapy.org

American Qigong Association
415-285-9400
www.eastwestqi.com

American Society for the Alexander Technique
800-473-0620
www.alexandertech.com

American Yoga Association
941-953-5859
www.americanyogaassociation.org

Association for Applied Psychophysiology and Biofeedback
303-422-8436
www.aapb.org

Biofeedback Certification Institute of America
303-420-2902
www.bcia.org

Center for Mind-Body Medicine
202-966-7338
www.cmbm.org

Certification Board for Nutrition Specialists
727-446-6086
www.cert-nutrition.org

Eye Movement Desensitization and Reprocessing (EMDR)
   International Organization
512-451-5200
www.emdria.org

Herb Research Foundation
1007 Pearl Street
Boulder, CO 80302
303-449-2262
www.herbs.org

International Taoist Tai Chi Society
416-656-2110
http://taoist.org

National Association of Cognitive Behavioral Therapists
800-853-1135
www.nacbt.org

National Certification Board for Therapeutic Massage and Bodywork
800-296-0664
www.ncbtmb.com

National Certification Commission for Acupuncture and Oriental Medicine
703-548-9004
www.nccaom.org

Somatic Experiencing
303-823-9524
www.traumahealing.org
Recommended contact: Yiri Dollekamp
212-586-1650
E-mail: yiri@aol.com

Stress Reduction Clinic
508-856-2656

NUTRITIONAL AND HERBAL SUPPLEMENT MANUFACTURERS AND DISTRIBUTORS

Advanced Nutritional Products
888-436-7200

Allergy Research Group
800-545-9960

Avena Botanicals
207-594-0694

Carlson Laboratories
888-234-5656

Country Life
631-231-1031

Davinci Laboratories
800-325-1776

Douglas Laboratories
888-DOUGLAB

Eclectic Institute
800-332-4372

Ecological Formulations, Inc.
Cardiovascular Research
800-888-4585

Enzymatic Therapy
920-469-1313

Gaia Herbs
800-831-7780

Genisoy Products
888-436-4769

Klaire Laboratories, Inc.
800-533-7255

Lane Labs
800-526-3005

Madis Botanicals
201-440-5000

Metagenics
800-338-3948

Nature's Herbs
800-437-2257

Nature's Way
801-489-1500

Nutra Soy
919-967-7261

Pure Encapsulations
800-753-CAPS

Scientific Botanicals
206-527-5521

Solgar Vitamin and Herb
877-765-4274

Thorne Research
800-228-1966

Twin Laboratories, Inc.
631-467-3140

Tyler Encapsulations
503-661-5401

Vitaline Formulas
800-648-4755

Index

Page numbers in italics indicate illustrations.

Aching muscles, statin drugs and, 28–29
Activities, stressful, 225
Acupuncture, 242–43, 255
Adams, Patch, *Gesundheit!*, 241
Additional supplementation, 3
　See also Nutritional supplements
Adenosine triphosphate (ATP), 54–55, 180
Adolescents, overweight, 62
Adrenal glands, and cholesterol, 19
Adult-onset diabetes (type 2), 33, 55–58, 62
　See also Diabetes
Advanced complicated atherosclerotic lesion, 13
Aerobic exercise, 207–8, 211–12, 219–23
Aflatoxin, 124
African-Americans, and hypertension, 48
Agar, 126
Age, as risk factor for CVD, 77, 83, 84, 88
Aging, 40, 48
　drug side effects and, 29
ALA (alpha-linolenic acid), 136–37
Alcohol, 52, 120
Allium, 45, 92
Alpha brain waves, 239
Alpha-linolenic acid (ALA), 136–37
Alpha-lipoic acid, 195
Alternative lifestyles, 254
Alternative medicine, 34–35
Alzheimer's disease, gingko biloba and, 197
American Dairy Council, 131
American Heart Association, 8, 18, 41, 52, 75
American Heart Institute, 20
Amino acids, 39, 95, 121–22

Anatomy of an Illness as Perceived by the Patient,
　Cousins, 241
Anemia, diet for, 148
Anerobic exercise, 209–10
Anger, 227–28
Angina pectoris, 15, 17, 31, 72
　supplements for, 197, 198–99
Angioplasty, 40
Animal-based proteins, 128–32
　customized diets, 143, 144, 145–46
Anti-fungal medications, and statin drugs, 31
Antibiotics
　and statin drugs, 31
　in animal products, 128–29
Antidepressants, exercise as, 208
Antioxidants, 71, 94, 95, 96, 99, 101–2, 109,
　　118–19, 174, 176–77, 187, 191, 192, 195
　statin drugs and, 31
Anxiety, 227
　exercise and, 208
Apolipoprotein B, 33
Apoproteins, 23, 37
Apoptosis (cell death), 13
Apples, 117
Arame, 126–27
Arginine, 186, 195
Aristotle, 206
Arrhythmias, 31, 200
Arteries, *14*
　inflammation of, 2
　plaque buildup and, 14–15
　See also Cardiovascular disease
Arthritis, turmeric and, 200

Art therapy, 237
Atherosclerosis, 8, 9, 11, 15
    fibrinogen and, 45
    homocysteine and, 38, 41
    obesity and, 66
Atorvastin (Lipitor), 247
ATP (adenosine triphosphate), 54–55, 180
Autonomy, and diet non-compliance, 252–53
Aviram, Michael, 120
Avocado, 134

Balloon angioplasty, 46, 182
Bananas, 117
Baycol (cerivastatin), 29–31, 34, 35
Benson, Herbert, 238, 240
Berries, 118–19
Beta-blockers, 215–16
Beta-carotene, 109, 116, 122, 131, 132, 134, 173
Beta-glucan, 113
Biaxin (clarithromycin), 194
Bicycle, stationary, 214–15
Bile acid sequestrants, 34
Biofeedback, 239–40
Biotin, 92, 122, 126, 131, 132, 134, 179
Birth control pills, 73, 78
    and diet, 148–49
Blood, 23, 37
    clotting of, 184
    flow of, obstructed, 8–16
Blood clot (thrombus), 13, *16,* 16
    homocysteine and, 40
    HRT and, 76
    insulin and, 60
Blood lipid profiles, 24–26
    NCEP-ATP III guidelines, 22
Blood pressure, 8, 10, 71
    orange juice and, 119
    supplements for, 198
    taurine and, 200
    See also Hypertension
Blood-sugar levels, 54
Blood tests, risk factors for CVD, 83
Blood-thinners, 13
    gingko biloba and, 197
    and statin drugs, 30, 31
    vitamin E as, 177–78
Body-based relaxation techniques, 242–43
Body fat, distribution of, 65
Body mass index (BMI), 62–64, 66, 84–85
Bodywork, 243
Bonow (cardiologist), 270
Boron, 174
Bran, 116
Breads, 114–15

Brillat-Savarin, Anthelme, 141
Broccoli, 109
Bromelain, 195–96
Bronchitis, chronic, 73
Brundtland, Gro Harlem, 271
Bypass surgery, 182, 187, 228

Calcium, 92–94, 109, 123, 125, 126, 127, 128, 131, 148, 174, 179–80, 183, 195
Calisthenics, 210
Campesterol, 111
Cancer, 8, 75
    hormone replacement therapy and, 76
    obesity and, 62
Canola oil, 135
Capsaicin, 94
Carbamezapine (Tegretol), 41, 78
Carbohydrates, 54, 117, 132–33, 146
    complex, 112, 116, 125
    USDA food pyramid and, 104
Carbon monoxide poisoning, 71–72
Cardiac-CRP, 43, 87
Cardiac insufficiency, 197–98
Cardiac output, 48
Cardiovascular disease (CVD), 1, 8–16, 17, 270
    cholesterol and, 20–21
    deaths from, 7–8, 20–21
    fibrates and, 33
    risk factors, 2, 3–4, 27, 36–37, 74–88
        C-reactive protein, 42–44
        diabetes, 53, 58–60
        elevated fibrinogen, 45
        elevated homocysteine, 38–42
        elevated lipoprotein (a), 45–46
        elevated triglycerides, 37–38
        hypertension, 47–52
        NCEP-ATP III and, 22
        obesity, 62–68
        sedentary lifestyle, 206–7
        smoking, 69–73
        stress, 224–45
CARE (coronary artery rehabilitation eating) diet, 45, 91, 271
    customized, 141–70
    food pyramid, *105,* 105–38
Carotenoids, 109, 110
Carroll, Lewis, 61
Catecholamines, 59
Celery, 148
Cell membranes, cholesterol and, 19
Cereals, 114, 150
Cerebral vascular accident. *See* Stroke
Cerivastatin (Baycol), 29–31, 34, 35
Chevreul, Michel Eugène, 19–20

Chicken soup, 130
Chick peas (garbanzo beans), 148, 149
Children, overweight, 62, 66
Chlamydia pneumoniae, 79
Cholesterol, 2, 9–10, 18–21, 22–24, 27, 66, 83
   diabetes and, 59
   exercise and, 208
   fats and, 133–38
   fiber and, 115–16
   guggulipid and, 188–89
   hypertension and, 50
   L-carnitine and, 198
   LDL, *11, 12,* 12–13
   measurement of, 24–26
   milk thistle and, 199
   niacin and, 183
   nuts and, 123–24
   oats and, 113
   oxidized, 13
   pantethine and, 199–200
   phytosterols and, 111–12
   policosanol and, 189–90
   red yeast rice and, 191–92
   and triglycerides, 38
   vitamin C and, 174–75
   vitamin E and, 176
Cholesterol-lowering drugs, 27–35
Cholestin, 193
Cholestyramine, 34
Choline, 94, 113, 132, 134, 179
Chromium, 94, 109, 113, 129, 131, 174
Chronic illness, and elevated homocysteine, 40
Cigarette smoke, 70–71
Circulation journal, 180, 270
Citrus fruits, 119
Clarithromycin (Biaxin), 194
Claudication. *See* Intermittent claudication
Cobalamin, 173
   See also Vitamins, B-complex
Coconut, 133–34
Coenzyme A, 199
Coenzyme Q$_{10}$, 31, 186–88, 194, 195
Cofactors, 40
Cohen, Jay, 35
Cold-water fish, 122–23
Colestipol (Colestid), 34, 41, 78
Collard greens, 149
Comfort foods, 251–52
Commiphora mukul (guggulipid), 188, 195
Community support, 243–44
Competitive sports, 219
Complex carbohydrates, 112, 116, 125
Condiments, serving sizes, 161
Congenital hyperhomocysteinemia, 38

Congestive heart failure, 17, 31, 49
   supplements for, 197–200
ConsumerLab.com, 203
Copper, 94, 113, 123, 174
Coronary artery disease, hypertension and, 49
   See also Cardiovascular disease
Costs
   of cardiovascular disease, 8
   of hypertension, 52
Coumarins, 94, 119, 123
Counseling for stress reduction, 235–36
Cousins, Norman, *Anatomy of an Illness as Perceived by the Patient,* 241
Cowper, William, 18
Cranberries, 118–19
Cravings, 254–55
C-reactive protein (CRP), 37, 42–44, 76
Cruciferous vegetables, 109
Curcuma longa (turmeric), 200–201
CVD. *See* Cardiovascular disease
Cyano-cobalamin, 101
Cyclosporin (Neoral, Sandimmune), 194
Cystathionine, 39
Cysteine, 39
Cytokines, 13, 66

Daily food diary, 257–58, *260*
Daily stress/relaxation log, 229–32
Dairy products, 131, 133–34, 143, 146, 159–60
   USDA food pyramid and, 104
Dance/movement therapy, 237
Dark green vegetables, 109
DEAR (Diet, Exercise, Additional supplementation, Relaxation) program, 3–4, 27, 32–33, 35, 52, 60, 82, 247, 271
Death, causes of, 7–8, 69–70, 75
Dehydroepiandrosterone (DHEA), 19
Department of Agriculture, U.S. (USDA), food pyramid, 102–5, *103*
Department of Health and Human Services, U.S. (HHS), 102
Depression, 227–29
DHA (docosahexaenoic acid), 122, 136–37
DHEA (dehydroepiandrosterone), 19
Diabetes, 50, 53–60, 62, 83, 85, 147, 208
   alpha lipoic acid and, 195
   beta-glucan and, 113–14
   and C-reactive protein, 43
   gestational, 57
   magnesium and, 180
   NCEP-ATP III and, 22
   niacin and, 185
   type 1 (juvenile onset), 55
   type 2 (adult-onset), 33, 55–58, 62

Diastolic blood pressure, 48
Diet, 3, 52, 91–140
    lack of compliance, 251–55
    record of, 257–58, *260*
Dietary Supplement Health and Education Act of 1994 (DSHEA), 202
Dietary supplements, FDA and, 201–2
    See also Nutritional supplements
Digitalis (Digoxin), 198
Diglyceride, 58
Dilantin (phenytoin), 41, 78
Diuretics, thiazide-based, 41
Docosahexaenoic acid (DHA), 122, 136–37
Dosages, 172–73
Drugs, cholesterol-lowering, 27–35
DSHEA (Dietary Supplement Health and Education Act of 1994), 202
Dulse, 127
Dysglycemia, 56

EBV (Epstein-Barr virus), 79
Edison, Thomas, 91
EDRF (endothelial derived relaxing factor), 75, 186
EFAs (essential fatty acids), 135–36, 181–83
Eggs, 131–34, 146, 159
Eicosapentaenoic acid (EPA), 45, 122, 136–37
Elagic acid, 139
EMDR (Eye movement desensitization and reprocessing), 237
Emphysema, 73
E-Mycin (erythromycin), 194
Endothelial derived relaxing factor (EDRF), 75, 186
Endothelial dysfunction, fibrinogen and, 45
Endothelium, damage to, 10, *10,* 40, 59, 70
    fatty deposits, 10–12, *11, 12*
    hypertension and, 50–51
Environmental toxins, 10
Enzyme deficiency, homocysteine and, 40
EPA (eicosapentaenoic acid), 45, 122, 136–37
Epetimibe (Zetia), 34
Epinephrine, 226
Epstein-Barr virus (EBV), 79
Erythromycin (E-Mycin, ERYC), 194
Essential amino acids, 39, 121–22
Essential fatty acids (EFAs), 135–37, 181–82, 183, 195
Estrogen, 19, 43, 75–76
Ethnicity
    and diabetes, 57
    and hypertension, 48
Exercise, 3, 22, 38, 52, 206–23, 271
    customized programs, 219–23
    daily record, 259, *261,* 262
    lack of, and C-reactive protein, 43
    poor tolerance, coenzyme Q_{10} and, 31
Exercise-based meditation, 241
Exercise pyramids, *220, 221, 222, 223, 261*
Eye movement desensitization and reprocessing (EMDR), 237

Family history, and CVD, 77–78, 83, 85
Farnesoid X receptor (FXR), 189
Fat cells, and endothelium, 10–12, *11, 12*
Fats, 133–38
    USDA food pyramid and, 104
Fatty streak, 11–13
FDA (Food and Drug Administration), 192–93, 201–2
Ferritin levels, 83, 84, 88
Fiber, dietary, 22, 108, 112–16, 123, 125, 126, 142
Fibrates, 28, 33–34
Fibrinogen, 37, 44–45, 70–71, 83, 84, 88
Fibrous cap, *12,* 13, 15
    rupture of, *16,* 16
Fight-or-flight response, 226–27
Figs, 119
Fish, 45, 121–23, 137, 155–56
Fish oil supplements, 181–82
Flavonoids, 95, 109, 116, 118, 119, 197–98
Foam cells, 11, *12,* 13, *16*
Folic acid (folate), 40, 41, 101, 110, 122, 125, 129, 130, 148–49, 174, 178–79, 183, 195
    See also Vitamins, B-complex
Fontaine, Jean de la, 47
Food cravings, 254–55
Food pyramid, 102–5, *103*
    CARE diet, *105,* 105–38
    high risk, *145*
    mild risk, *142*
    moderate risk, *143*
Framingham Disability Study, 20, 73, 209
Frankl, Viktor, 245
Free radicals, 40, 59, 70–71, 138, 175
Friendships, 244
Fruit juices, 107, 121, 154
Fruits, 104, 106, 117–21, 142, 153–55
    USDA food pyramid and, 104
FXR (farnesoid X receptor), 189

Gallstones, cholesterol and, 19–20
Game (wild meat), 129
Gamma-linolenic acid (GLA), 136
Gangrene, in diabetes, 59
Garbanzo beans (chick peas), 148, 149
Garlic, 45, 197
Gemfibrozil (Lopid), 31, 193–94

Gender
  and elevated homocysteine, 41
  and risk of CVD, 74–77, 83, 86
Genetic factors
  in cardiovascular disease, 77–78
  in diabetes, 55, 57
  in elevated lipoprotein (a), 46
Genistein, 95
Gestational diabetes, 57
Gesundheit!, Adams, 241
Ginger, 139
Ginkgo biloba, 196–97
GLA (gamma-linolenic acid), 136
Global Embrace, 270–71
Global risk assessment, 82
Glucagon, 54–55
Glucose, 54–57
Glucose intolerance, 56
Glutathione, 95, 109, 116–17, 119, 195
Glycerides, 57
Glycogen, 54–56
Good Housekeeping Institute, 203
Grapefruit juice, and statin drugs, 30
Grapes, 119–20
Grapeseed extract, 197
Green leafy vegetables, 137, 148, 149
Green tea, 139
Grinkov, Sergei, 81–82
Growth hormones in animal products, 129
Guggulipid (*Commiphora mukul*), 188, 195
Guided imagery, 255
Guidelines for blood components, 21–22
  See also NCEP-ATP III guidelines

Habit, and diet non-compliance, 253–54
Harvard Medical School, 38
Hawthorn, 197–98
HDL (high-density lipoprotein) cholesterol, 21, 22–26, 57, 87
  See also Cholesterol
Healing, planetary, 271
Health club membership, 215
Heart, 7
  diseases of. *See* Cardiovascular disease
Heart and Estrogen/Progestin Replacement Study (HERS), 76
Heart attack, 8, 16, 17, 45, 46, 51, 76
  depression and, 228
Heavy metals, 10, 122
Helicobacter pylori, 79, 109
Herpes virus, 79, 186
HERS (Heart and Estrogen/Progestin Replacement Study), 76

HHS (Health and Human Services Department, U.S.), 102
High blood pressure, 10, 31, 47–52
  diet for, 148
  See also Hypertension
High risk status
  customized CARE diet, 144–46
  daily menus, 168–69
  exercise program, 222–23, *223*
  nutritional supplements, 194–201
High-sensitivity CRP (hs-CRP), 43
Hijiki, 127
HMG-CoA reductase, 28, 189–90, 191, 194
Holistic medicine, 3, 27, 34–35
Homeostasis, 58
Homocysteine, 10, 37, 38–42, 83, 87
  vitamin C and, 175
  vitamin E and, 176
Homocysteinuria, 38
Hormone replacement therapy (HRT), 76
Hormones, cholesterol and, 19
Hs-CPR (high-sensitivity CPR), 43, 83
Hu, Frank, 56
Hydrocarbons, 70
Hydrogenated fats, 137–38, 146
Hypercalcemia, 181
Hyperhomocysteinemia, congenital, 38
Hypertension, 2, 47–52, 83, 85
  calcium and, 180
  diabetes and, 57, 60
  exercise and, 208
  obesity and, 62, 66
  smoking and, 71
Hypnosis, 255

Illness, and elevated homocysteine, 41
Immune cells, 9, 11–13
Independence, and diet non-compliance, 252–53
Inderal (propranolol), 216
Indoles, 95–96, 109
Infections, 10, 41, 79–80, 83, 84, 88
  and C-reactive protein, 42, 43
Inflammation, 2, 9, 16, 80
  bromelain and, 196
  C-reactive protein and, 42
  essential fatty acids and, 136
  exercise and, 208
  fibrinogen and, 44
  HRT and, 76
  obesity and, 66
  supplements for, 197
  turmeric and, 200–201
Inflammatory response, 9
Inositol, 94, 113, 132, 134, 174, 179

Inositol hexanicotinate, 185
Insoluble fiber, 115
Insulin, 54–56
Insulin resistance, 33, 50, 56, 57–58, 59–60, 83, 85, 180, 199
   See also Diabetes
Intensity of exercise, 215–16
Intermittent claudication, 15, 72, 190
   supplements for, 197, 198
Internal stressors, 226–27
International Day of Older Persons, 271
Iodine, 126, 127, 174
Iron, 96, 109, 113, 125, 126, 127, 128, 129, 130, 148
Ischemia, 72
Isoflavones, 96, 191
Isolation, social, 228, 243–44
Isoprenyl, 186

Juvenile-onset (type 1) diabetes, 55

Kelp, 127
Kidney damage, hypertension and, 51
Kile, Darryl, 82
Kombu, 127

Lamb, 129, 149
L-arginine, 186
Laughter, 241–42
L-carnitine, 198–99, 255
LDL (low-density lipoprotein) cholesterol, 11, *12*, 12–13, 21, 22–26, 86, 107
   berries and, 118
   fibrates and, 33
   lipoprotein (a), 45–46
   NCEP-ATP III guidelines, 22
   See also Cholesterol
Lecithin, 132
Leeks, 137
Legumes, 125, 149, 156–57
Lesion, in blood vessel, 12–15, *12, 14*
Leukocytes (white blood cells), 11, 12, 13
Levine, Peter A., 238
Lieberman, Shari, 114
Lifestyle
   alterations, 32
      to reduce stress, 232–34
   and blood-pressure control, 52
   and diabetes, 56–57
   exercise programs and, 213–23
   heart-healthy, and plaque, 15
   risk factors for CVD, 83
   sedentary, 43, 68, 79, 83, 206–7, 210–11
Lignans, 96, 112, 124

Lipid (fatty substance), cholesterol as, 19
Lipitor (atorvastin), 247
Lipoproteins, 23, 87
   Lp(a), 37, 45–46, 83
Liver
   alpha lipoic acid and, 195
   and cholesterol, 18–19, 23
   C-reactive protein manufacture, 42
   fibrates and, 33
   milk thistle and, 199
   statin drugs and, 28, 30
   triglyceride manufacture, 37
Long-chain alcohols, 189
Lopid (gemfibrozil), 31, 34, 193–94
Lopressor (metoprolol), 215–16
Lovastatin, 191
Love, 245
   of self, 3, 271
Lp(a). See Lipoproteins
Lumen, *14*, 15
Lycopene, 96, 119

McCully, Kilmer, 38
Macrophages (white blood cells), 11, *12*, 12
Macular degeneration, taurine and, 200
Magnesium, 97, 113, 117, 122, 123, 125, 127, 128, 174, 179–80, 183, 195
Manganese, 97, 174
Margarine, 134, 137–38
Martial arts, 241
Massage, 243
Measurement of cholesterol levels, 24–26
Meats, 129–30, 133–34, 158–59
Medications, 78
   cholesterol-lowering, 27–35
   and depression, 229
   and elevated homocysteine, 41
   smoking and, 73
   supplements and, 204
Meditation, 240–41
Mediterranean diet, 135
Memory loss, statin drugs and, 28–29
Menopause, 76, 148
   See also Postmenopausal women
Menus, 162–69
Mercury, in fish, 122
Meta-analysis, of homocysteine, 38–39
Metabolic syndrome. See Syndrome X
Methionine, 39
Methotrexate (Rheumatrex), 41, 78
Metoprolol (Lopressor), 215–16
Mild risk status
   customized CARE diet, 141–43
   daily menus, 164–65

exercise program, 220–21, *221*
nutritional supplements, 174–82
Milk thistle (*Silibum marianum*), 199
Minerals, 92–94, 96, 97, 98–99, 102
multivitamin supplement, 174, 182, 194
Moderate risk status
customized CARE diet, 143–44
daily menus, 166–67
exercise program, 221–22, *222*
nutritional supplements, 182–94
Monacolins, 191
Monascus purpureus, 191
Monocytes, *12,* 12
Monoglyceride, 58
Monoglycerol, 58
Mononucleosis, 79
Monosaturated fatty acids, 123, 135, 191
Mono-unsaturated fats, 124
Motivation, lack of, 246–48
Multiple Risk Factor Intervention Trial (MRFIT), 20, 210–11
Multivitamin and mineral supplement, 173–74, 182, 194
Muscle enzymes, test of, 30
Muscle mass, loss of, 67–68
Muscle tissue, statin drugs and, 28
Mushrooms, 109–10
Music therapy, 237
Mycoplasma pneumoniae, 79
Myocardial infarction, 8

National Cholesterol Education Program. *See* NCEP
National Health and Nutrition Examination Survey (NHANES) III, 52, 66
National Institute of Diabetes and Digestive and Kidney Diseases (NIDDK), 62
National Institutes of Health (NIH), 20–21, 62
Native Americans, fibrinogen study, 45
NCEP (National Cholesterol Education Program), 21
ATP III guidelines, 2, 22, 27, 32
and obesity, 66–67
diabetes as risk factor, 53
triglycerides, 37–38
phytosterols, 111–12
Necrosis (decay of dead tissue), 13, 59
Necrotic core, 13
Neoral (cyclosporin), 194
Nerves
cholesterol and, 19, 23
statin drugs and, 28
Neurology journal, 28
Neurotransmitters, 39

Niacin, 46, 100, 127, 179, 183–84, 193, 195
See also Vitamins, B-complex
Niacinamide, 179, 183
See also Vitamins, B-complex
Niacor, Niaspan (nicotinic acid), 41
Nicotine, 70, 71
Nicotinic acid (Niacor, Niaspan), and elevated homocysteine, 41
NIH (National Institutes of Health), 62
Nonessential amino acids, 200
Nonfat dairy products, 144
Nonstarchy vegetables, 104, 108–11, 151–52
customized diets, 142, 144, 145
Nonverbal therapies, 236–38
Norepinephrine, 226
Nori, 127–28
NSF International, 203
Nurses' Study, 210
Nutrients, 92–102
Nutritional supplements, 171–205
daily record, 259, 263–67
resources, 296–98
Nuts, 122–23, 134, 135, 137, 157–58

Oats, 113
Obesity, 43, 61–68, 83, 84–85, 208
diabetes and, 57, 60
Oils, 104, 134–35
Old age, 40, 83
Olive oil, 45, 135, 137
Omega-3 fatty acids, 122, 135–37, 255
Omega-6 fatty acids, 135–36
Onions, 45, 109
Oral contraceptives, 78, 148–49
Orange juice, 119
Organically grown foods, 128–29, 131
Ornish, Dean, 32
Osteoporosis, 179, 209
Overdosage, 35
Overprescription of statin drugs, 2
Overweight, 62–63, 149
Oxidized cholesterol, 13

PABA (para-amino-benzoic acid), 97, 109, 113, 132, 134, 174, 179
Pacemaker cells, 77
Pancreas, malfunction of, 54, 58
See also Diabetes
Pantethine, 199–200
Pantothenic acid, 100–101, 109, 174, 199–200
See also Vitamins, B-complex
Para-amino-benzoic acid. *See* PABA
Paraoxonase, 120
Pasta, 116

Peanuts, 124, 125
Pectin, 117, 118, 119
Periodontal disease, 80, 118, 187
Peripheral artery disease, 17
Peripheral neuropathy, statin drugs and, 28
Peripheral resistance, 48
Peripheral vascular disease, 38
  smoking and, 72
Personal history, risk factors for CVD, 83, 85
Personal workbook, 256–69
Personality
  type A, 83, 227, 229
  type D, 228, 229
Pesticide residues in animal products, 129
Pharmanex, 193
Phenols, 118
Phenytoin (Dilantin), 41, 78
Phosphorus, food sources, 98, 113, 122–32, 134
Physical activity, 38
Physicians' Health Study II, 45
Phytochemicals, 125
Phytoestrogens, 95, 96, 148
Phyto-feasting tips, 146–47
Phytonutrients, 92, 94–96, 98, 108, 142
Phytosterols, 111–12
Pinto beans, 137
Plant-based proteins, 106, 123–28
Plant stanols, 111–12
Plaque, 8, 9–10, 11, *12,* 13–15, 44
  cholesterol and, 23–24, 27
  diabetes and, 59
  hypertension and, 50
  stable, lifestyle and, 15
  unstable, 16, 81
Platelets, 13
Policosanol, 189–90, 193, 195
Polyphenols, 98, 109, 123
Polyunsaturated fats, 134
Pomegranates, 120
Pork, 129, 149
Postmenopausal women, risk of CVD, 44, 76–77, 83, 86
Potassium, food sources, 98, 116, 117, 119, 124, 125, 126, 127
Potatoes, 116
Poultry, 130, 133–34, 143, 158–59
Prayer, 245
Preclinical atherosclerosis, 45
Pregnenolone, 19
Preventive diet, daily menus, 162–63
Preventive exercise program, 219–20, *220*
Proanthocyanidins, 197
Progesterone, 19
Propranolol (Inderal), 216

Prostaglandins, 136, 183–84
Protease inhibitors, 194
Proteins, 39, 106, 121–23
  animal-based, 128–32
  plant-based, 123–28
Psychotherapy, 235–36
Pulse rates, target, 215–16
Purslane, 137
Pyridoxine, 101, 173

Qigong, 241
Quinones, 186
Qureshi, Asaf A., 113–14

Rational dosing, 35
Red wine, 45, 119–20
Red yeast rice, 190–94, 195
Relaxation, 3, 238–43
  daily record, 268–69
Relaxation response, 238–40
Religion, 245
Remodeling of artery, *14,* 14–15
Reproductive organs, and cholesterol, 19
Resorption, 179
Resources, 291–98
Restenosis, 40, 46, 175
Resveratrol, 119
Rhabdomyolysis, 29, 33–34
Rheumatoid arthritis, 42
Rheumatrex (methotrexate), 78, 41
Riboflavin, 100, 109, 173, 179
Rice bran, 113–14
Ridker, Paul, 79–80
Risk of CVD, assessment of, 81–84
  Risk-Factor Questionnaire, 84–88
Roberts, William, 29
Root vegetables, 116

Salmon, 45
Sandimmune (cyclosporin), 194
Saponins, 98–99
Saturated fat, 128, 133–34
Scavenger cells. *See* Macrophages
Schweitzer, Albert, 224
Sea vegetables, 126–28, 146–47, 148, 156
Sedentary lifestyle, 79, 83, 86, 206–7, 210–11
Seeds, 124–25, 134, 137, 158
Selenium, 99, 109, 113, 122, 174
Self, love of, 3, 271
Self-care, obstacles to, 246–55
Serving sizes, 150–61
Sex hormones, cholesterol and, 19, 23
Shakespeare, William, 7, 36, 53
Shallots, 45

Shapiro, Francine, 237
Shellfish, serving sizes, 155–56
Shiatsu, 243
Side effects of medications, 1, 28–31, 33
Sidney, Philip, 256
Siegel, Bernie, 3, 242
Silibim marianum (milk thistle), 199
Sitostanol, 111
Sitosterol, 111–12
Sleep, 234–35, 239
Smoking, 41, 43, 52, 69–73, 83, 84
Smooth muscle cells, *11, 12,* 13
Social aspects of diet, 254
Social connection, 243–44
Sodas, 107
Sodium, 99, 148
Solid organ transplantation, 41
Soluble fiber, 115
Somatic experiencing, 238
Soy products, 137, 148
Sphygmomanometer, 48
Spirituality, 245
Spreads, serving sizes, 161
Sprouts, 109, 142, 144, 145
Standardized extract, 203
Starchy foods, 103–4
Starchy vegetables, 104, 106, 116–17, 155
Statin drugs, 1, 2, 27–33, 99, 109, 136, 195
    coenzyme Q_{10} and, 187
    milk thistle and, 199
    niacin and, 184–86
    red yeast rice and, 191
Stationary bicycle, 214–15
Sterols, in red yeast rice, 191
Stews, 149
Stigmasterol, 111
Stomach ulcers, 79
Storage of supplements, 204–5
Strawberries, 119
Strength-building exercise, 209–10
Stress, 79, 83–84, 88, 224–29
    daily record, 268–69
    reduction of, 52, 229–46
Stretching, 210, 217, 219
Stroke, 8, 16, 17, 38, 73, 75, 196
    diabetes and, 59
    HRT and, 78
    hypertension and, 50, 51
Strong Heart Study, 45
Sugars, 38, 54, 57, 117, 132–33
Sulfites, 120, 124
Sulfur, 99, 109
Sulfurophane, 109
Summer squash, 110

Sunlight, 180
Syndrome X (metabolic syndrome), 2, 21, 22, 36
    diabetes and, 60
    hypertension and, 50
    obesity and, 66
Systolic blood pressure, 48

Tai chi, 241
Taking of supplements, 204
Target pulse rates, 215–16
Taurine, 200
Tea, 139
Tegretol (carbamezapine), 41, 78
Testosterone, 19, 75
Tests
    before exercise programs, 212
    for cholesterol levels, 24–26
    for C-reactive protein, 43–44
    for homocysteine levels, 41–42
TFA (transfatty acid), 137–38
Therapeutic lifestyle changes (TLC), 22
Thiamin, 100, 173, 179
    See also Vitamins, B-complex
Thiazide diuretics, 41, 78
Thirst, as symptom of diabetes, 58
Thompson, Francis, 69
Thrombus. *See* Blood clot
Time, lack of, 248–50
TLC (therapeutic lifestyle changes), 22
Tobacco. *See* Smoking
Tocopherols, 176
Tocotrienols, 176–77
Tofu, 146
Transcendental Meditation (TM), 240
Transfatty acid (TFA), 137–38
Treadmill, 214–15
Triglycerides, 36, 37–38, 57–58, 59–60, 83, 88
    bile acid sequestrants, and, 34
    and diabetes, 57
    exercise and, 208
    fibrates and, 33
    guggulipid and, 188
    hypertension and, 50
    L-carnitine and, 198–99
    NCEP-ATP III guidelines, 22
    niacin and, 183
    pantethine and, 200
    policosanol and, 190
Turmeric (*Curcuma longa*), 200–201

Ubiquinone, 186–88
    See also Coenzyme Q_{10}

United States Pharmacopoeia (USP), 203
Unstable plaque, 81
USDA (U.S. Department of Agriculture), food pyramid, 102–5, *103*
USP (United States Pharmacopoeia), 203

Valvular heart disease, 17
Vanadium, 99, 113, 132, 134
Vasculitis, C-reactive protein and, 42
Vasoconstrictor, cigarette smoke as, 71
Vegetables, 104, 106, 147
    nonstarchy, 108–11
    USDA food pyramid and, 104
Very low-density lipoprotein (VLDL), 33, 37, 60, 183
Vinson, Joe, 118
Viruses, damage to endothelium, 10
Vitamins, 34, 41, 45, 92, 94, 97, 99, 116, 174–81, 194–95
    A, 99, 109, 110, 116, 122, 126, 127, 128, 131, 132, 134, 173
    B-complex, 40, 92, 94, 97, 100–101, 113, 122, 123, 124, 125, 126, 127, 128, 129, 130, 131, 132, 134, 178–79, 183, 195, 199–200
    C, 45, 46, 101–2, 109, 118, 119, 127, 128, 174–76, 182, 194
    D, 127, 174, 179–81
    E, 45, 99, 102, 109, 113, 117, 123, 127, 132, 134, 174, 176–78, 182, 195, 201
    K, 102, 109
    multivitamin supplement, 173–74
VLDL. *See* Very low-density lipoprotein
Volunteering, 244

Wakame, 128
Walking, 210, 213–14, 216, 218
    meditation, 241
Walnuts, 123–24
Water, 106–7
Website, 4
Weekly exercise diary, *262*
Weight control, 38
Weight loss, 22, 52, 67–68, 149, 208
Weight training, 209
White blood cell count, and death from heart attack, 16
White blood cells. *See* Leukocytes
Whitecoat hypertension, 48
White-flour products, 104, 132–33, 160
Whole grains, 106, 112–16, 152–53
    customized diets, 142, 144, 145
Whole wheat, 149
Wild game, 129
Willett, Walter, 105
Williams, Robin, 241
Willpower, lack of, 250–51
Winter squash, 116–17
Women's Health Initiative, 76
Workbook, 256–69
World Health Organization (WHO), 8
World Heart Day, 270–71
World Heart Federation, 270

Yeast, 149
Yoga, 241
Yo-yo dieting, 67

Zetia (epetimibe), 34